Lecture Notes in Bioengineering

Lecture Notes in Bioengineering (LNBE) publishes the latest developments in bioengineering. It covers a wide range of topics, including (but not limited to):

- Bio-inspired Technology & Biomimetics
- Biosensors
- Bionanomaterials
- Biomedical Instrumentation
- Biological Signal Processing
- Medical Robotics and Assistive Technology
- Computational Medicine, Computational Pharmacology and Computational Biology
- Personalized Medicine
- Data Analysis in Bioengineering
- Neuroengineering
- Bioengineering Ethics

Original research reported in proceedings and edited books are at the core of LNBE. Monographs presenting cutting-edge findings, new perspectives on classical fields or reviewing the state-of-the art in a certain subfield of bioengineering may exceptionally be considered for publication. Alternatively, they may be redirected to more specific book series. The series' target audience includes advanced level students, researchers, and industry professionals working at the forefront of their fields.

Indexed by SCOPUS and Springerlink. The books of the series are submitted for indexing to Web of Science.

More information about this series at http://www.springer.com/series/11564

Anubha Gupta · Ritu Gupta
Editors

ISBI 2019 C-NMC Challenge: Classification in Cancer Cell Imaging

Select Proceedings

Springer

Editors
Anubha Gupta
IIIT Delhi
New Delhi, India

Ritu Gupta
Laboratory Oncology
AIIMS
New Delhi, India

ISSN 2195-271X ISSN 2195-2728 (electronic)
Lecture Notes in Bioengineering
ISBN 978-981-15-0797-7 ISBN 978-981-15-0798-4 (eBook)
https://doi.org/10.1007/978-981-15-0798-4

This Springer imprint is published by the registered company Springer Nature Singapore Pte Ltd.
The registered company address is: 152 Beach Road, #21-01/04 Gateway East, Singapore 189721, Singapore

Preface

This book contains proceedings of the medical image classification challenge, titled "C-NMC challenge: Classification of Normal versus Malignant Cells in B-ALL White Blood Cancer Microscopic Image" organized by researchers of SBILab, IIIT-Delhi (http://sbilab.iiitd.edu.in/), and AIIMS, New Delhi, India, as part of the IEEE International Symposium on Biomedical Imaging (IEEE-ISBI 2019) conference held in Venice, Italy, from April 8 to 11, 2019.

Cell classification via image processing has recently gained interest from the point of view of building computer-assisted diagnostic tools for blood disorders such as leukemia. In order to arrive at a conclusive decision on disease diagnosis and degree of progression, it is very important to identify malignant cells with high accuracy. Computer-assisted tools can be very helpful in automating the process of cell segmentation and identification because morphologically both cell types appear similar. This challenge was run on a curated dataset of more than 15000 cell images of very good quality.

The challenge had participants from many countries. The training data was provided to 251 teams, and the number of submissions on the preliminary test data and the final test data on the challenge leaderboard was 60 and 25, respectively. The challenge was opened on November 10, 2018, at CodaLab, and the results were declared on March 18, 2019. The results of the challenge on the test set predictions are available at the challenge leaderboard (http://sbilab.iiitd.edu.in/resources.html). The challenge concluded with a workshop at IEEE-ISBI 2019 conference on April 11, 2019, wherein three top performing teams and five other teams presented their work. The challenge was technically co-sponsored by IBM India Pvt. Ltd. On behalf of IBM India, Dr. Mani Madhukar, Program Manager, University Relations, IBM India Pvt. Ltd, attended the workshop, delivered a lecture on IBM Watson, and also distributed the prizes to the top three teams as well as to the other participants of the challenge.

The dataset provided for this challenge, named *C-NMC 2019 Dataset*, was prepared at Laboratory Oncology, AIIMS, New Delhi, India. A waiver for written informed consent was obtained from the Ethics Committee of AIIMS, New Delhi, on this dataset for research purposes. It consisted of white blood cell images with labels (normal versus cancer) that were provided to train machine learning-based classifier to identify normal cells from leukemic blasts (malignant/cancer cells). This dataset is now publicly available at The Cancer Imaging Archive (TCIA) (https://doi.org/10.7937/tcia.2019.dc64i46r). Data is prepared at the subject level and is split into the training set and testing set. Training set consists of 12528 cell images collected from the data of 60 cancer subjects and 41 healthy subjects. Test data consists of 2586 cell images collected from 9 cancer subjects and 8 healthy subjects. The size of the total dataset is 15114 cell images. Researchers can evaluate their results on the test set by submitting results at the leaderboard (https://competitions.codalab.org/competitions/20395#results).

We gratefully acknowledge the research funding support (Grant: EMR/2016/006183) from the Department of Science and Technology, Govt. of India, and Grant: 1(7)/2014-ME\&HI from the Ministry of Communication and IT, Govt. of India, for this research work. The funder had no role in study design, data collection and analysis, decision to publish, or preparation of the manuscript. We acknowledge the support of IBM India Pvt. Limited for being the technical co-sponsor of this challenge. We are grateful to the Technical Program Committee, who devoted their valuable time in reviewing the submitted papers and provided constructive feedback to the authors. Each paper was reviewed by three independent reviewers. We thank all the workshop attendees who presented their work at the workshop in Venice. In particular, we would like to thank Shiv Gehlot, PhD Scholar, SBILab, Department of ECE, IIIT-Delhi, for handling the work related to challenge from start to the end. He helped participants with all their queries, maintained the challenge portal, helped participants evaluate the performance of their codes, and provided support for the publication of this challenge proceedings. Last but not least, we would like to thank the students and staff of SBILab, IIIT-Delhi, and Laboratory Oncology, AIIMS, New Delhi, for their support for the smooth conduct of this challenge and publications of the proceedings.

New Delhi, India

Anubha Gupta
Ritu Gupta

Contents

About the Editors

Dr. Anubha Gupta received her PhD in Electrical Engineering from Indian Institute of Technology (IIT) Delhi in 2006. She completed her second Master's as a full time student from the University of Maryland, College Park, USA from 2008-2010 in education with concentration: Higher Education Leadership and Policy Studies. She worked as Assistant Director with the Ministry of Information and Broadcasting, Government of India (through Indian Engineering Services) from 1993 to 1999 and as faculty for about 10 years before joining IIIT Delhi in December 2013, where she is currently working as Professor. She has author/co-authored over 80 technical papers in scientific journals and conferences. She has also filed 4 patents. She has published research papers in both engineering and education. Her research interests include biomedical signal and image processing including fMRI, MRI, DTI, EEG, ECG signal processing, genomics signal processing in cancer research, wavelets in deep learning, and signal processing for communication engineering. Dr. Gupta is a senior member of IEEE Signal processing Society, a member of IEEE Women in Engineering Society, and is Associate Editor of IEEE Access journal.

Dr. Ritu Gupta is Professor of Laboratory Oncology at the All India Institute of Medical Sciences (AIIMS), New Delhi. She is currently spearheading the cancer laboratories at Dr. B.R. Ambedkar IRCH, AIIMS and is actively engaged in establishing diagnostic and research laboratories at the National Cancer Institute (NCI), Jhajjar, India. Dr. Gupta and her research group have established Unit of Excellence on Multiple Myeloma at AIIMS. Her lab is investigating the genomic and epigenomic alterations responsible for disease progression and treatment response in chronic lymphocytic leukemia and the molecular basis of disease heterogeneity in multiple myeloma. She is also establishing a Center of Advanced research and Eduaction on Acute Myeloid Leukemia, the focus of which is the 'Leukemic Stem Cells'. As a hematopathologist, she has a keen interest in digital processing of tumor cells and is working on image processing based software solutions for clinical applications. She has published more than 90 papers in peer reviewed journals and is actively engaged in academic activities at the national level for training of medical fraternity on advanced laboratory diagnostics including multi-parametric flow cytometry and molecular assays for clinical diagnostics and research.

Classification of Normal Versus Malignant Cells in B-ALL White Blood Cancer Microscopic Images

Atmika Honnalgere and Gaurav Nayak

Abstract Identification of malignant cells is an important aspect of cancer diagnosis and in determining the degree of progression. Blood disorders, such as leukemia, are most often detected only in advanced stages, when the number of cancer cells is much higher than the number of normal cells. Differentiation of cancer cells from normal blood cells is challenging due to their acute morphological similarity. Early diagnosis of leukemia relies on the accurate classification of malignant cells versus normal cells in microscopic images of blood cells. Computer-aided cell classification has gained popularity as an efficient technique for the diagnosis of leukemia. Our approach to classification involves finetuning of a VGG16 neural network with batch normalization to classify the images of malignant vis-à-vis normal cells.

Keywords VGG16 · Transfer learning

1 Introduction

Leukemia is a group of blood cancers, which starts at the bone marrow and leads to the production of many abnormal blood cells. These cells are referred to as blasts.

The suspected causes of leukemia are varied. Genetic and environmental factors, smoking, prolonged exposure to ionizing radiation or chemicals, such as benzene, chemotherapy, and Down's syndrome are considered high risk factors.

Leukemia can be classified into four major types: acute lymphoblastic leukemia (ALL), acute myeloid leukemia (AML), chronic lymphocytic leukemia (CLL), and chronic myeloid leukemia (CML).

Diagnosis of leukemia is typically done through blood tests or bone marrow biopsy. Detection of blood disorders, such as leukemia, mostly occurs in advanced

A. Honnalgere (✉)
Occipital Tech, Mumbai 400703, India
e-mail: atmikah@gmail.com

G. Nayak
Indian Institute of Science, Bangalore 560012, India
e-mail: gauravnayak@iisc.ac.in

A. Gupta and R. Gupta (eds.), *ISBI 2019 C-NMC Challenge: Classification in Cancer Cell Imaging*, Lecture Notes in Bioengineering,
https://doi.org/10.1007/978-981-15-0798-4_1

stages, when malignant cells are present in greater number as compared to their numbers in a normal person. The ability to differentiate between malignant cells and normal cells is critical in diagnosing these blood disorders in their early stages.

Computer-aided diagnostic tools for leukemia have attracted great interest as a means for early prognosis. Cell classification via image processing has gained traction as a way to diagnose leukemia and determine its level of progression. It is a cheap and easily deployable method for diagnosis. However, the task of differentiating between malignant and normal cells is challenging due to their morphological similarities.

The paper is structured as follows: Sect. 2 discusses prior work done on the subject of leukemic cell classification. Section 3 describes our approach. Section 4 presents the observations gathered from our approach. Section 5 provides the results for the classification performed on the preliminary and final test dataset. Section 6 presents the conclusions drawn from the observations along with the possible improvement to our approach.

2 Previous Works

Krishna Kanth [1] proposes the fuzzy hyper sphere neural network (FHSNN) classifier for the discrimination of ALL and AML subtypes present in the blood cancer dataset. Since the number of genes is larger in number compared to the samples which are available in the microarray datasets, dimensionality reduction methods, such as signal-to-noise ratio (SNR), class-separability, Wilcoxon rank sum statistic, and Fisher ratio, are applied to the dataset before training. The experimental results show that FHSNN achieves 100% accuracy with less number of genes than the previously published methods. Adjouadi et al. [2] present a novel artificial neural network (ANN) algorithm for optimizing the classification of multidimensional data, focusing on the classification of abnormal versus normal blood samples, namely ALL and AML. This algorithm achieved an accuracy of up to 96.67% in ALL classification. Krishna Kanth et al. [3] propose a modification to FHSNN, known as modified fuzzy hyper sphere neural network (MFHSNN), for the discrimination of ALL and AML in blood cancer dataset. Dimensionality reduction methods, such as Spearman correlation coefficient and Wilcoxon rank sum test, are used for gene selection. A classification accuracy of 100% has been achieved using the MFHSNN classifier using only two genes. Amin et al. [4] discuss a method to distinguish acute lymphoblastic blood cancer cells from normal cells. After applying image preprocessing to the microscopic images of blood cells, cell nuclei are categorized by k-means algorithm. Geometric and statistical features are extracted from nuclei to classify them using support vector machine.

All these approaches use dimensionality reduction or special network architectures to process the dataset. Our approach is to use a convolutional neural network, which uses shared weights (kernels), thereby reducing computation. Furthermore, our approach reduces the time required to train the network by starting with a pretrained network and re-training it for leukemic blasts versus normal cell classification.

3 Approach

Our approach is to use transfer learning to adapt a VGG16 neural network with batch normalization, pretrained on the ImageNet dataset, to classify malignant and normal cells (Figs. 1 and 2).

VGG16. VGG16 [5] is a convolutional neural network (CNN) architecture developed by the Visual Geometry Group at Oxford University to compete with the ImageNet Large Scale Visual Recognition Challenge (ILSVRC) [6]. The ImageNet [7] dataset consists of 14,197,122 images across 1000 different categories of objects. The goal of the challenge is to train a model on the ImageNet dataset to correctly classify input

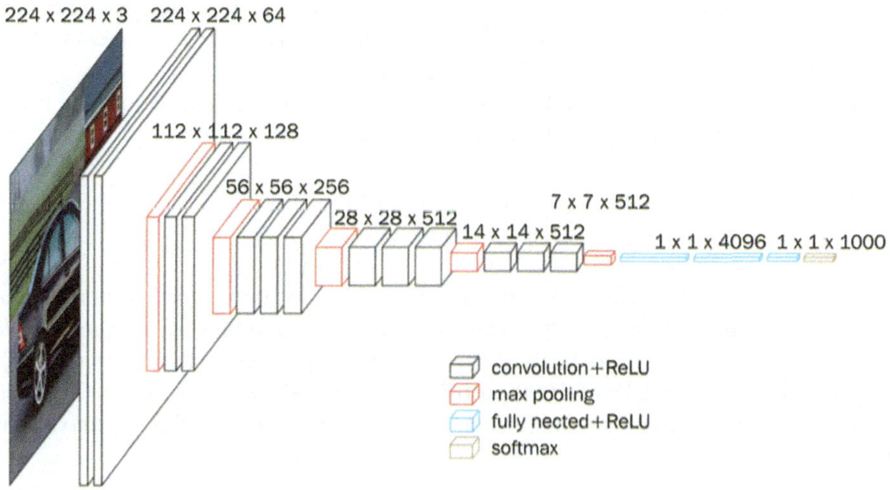

Fig. 1 Architecture of VGG16

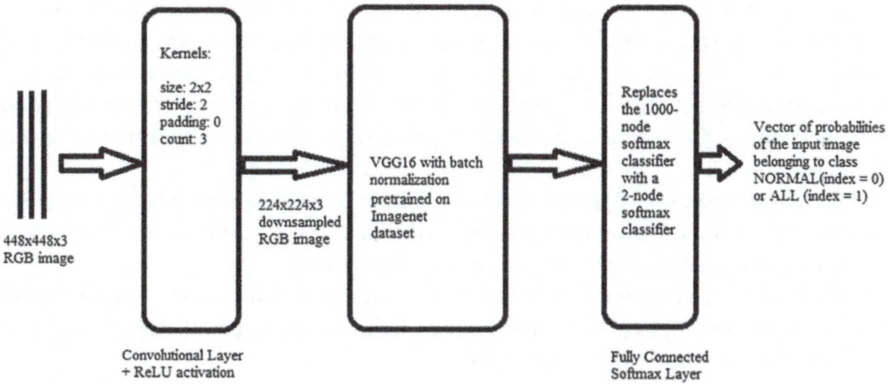

Fig. 2 Modified VGG16 architecture

images into 1000 classes present in the ImageNet dataset. VGG16 won ILSVRC in 2014.

The network has a simplistic design and only uses kernels of size 3 × 3 in convolutional layers that are stacked on top of each other. The stacking allows the network to capture greater information with lesser computational overhead. For example, three stacked convolutional layers with kernels of size 3 × 3 produce feature maps equivalent to one convolutional layer with kernels of size 7 × 7, with lesser computational overhead.

The max-pooling layers consist of kernels of size 2 × 2 which downsample the input by a factor of 2 by passing the maximum value in a neighborhood of 2 × 2 to the output. The input volume is reduced by factor of 4.

The networks end with two fully connected layers, each with 4096 nodes, followed by a 1000-node softmax classifier. The fully connected layers connect each node in the layer to every feature element in the input. These fully connected layers restrict the network input to a fixed size of 224 × 224 × 3.

The softmax classifier is a fully connected layer which applied the softmax function (σ) to the output features of the fully connected layer.

$$\sigma(z)_j = e^z_j / \Sigma_k e^z_k$$
$$\text{for } j = 1, \ldots, K \text{ and } z = (z_1, \ldots, z_K)$$

where z is the output feature vector of size K. The softmax function normalizes the output feature vector into a probability distribution, and produces a vector of K probabilities, that sum to 1. Each element of the output lies in the interval [0, 1]. VGG16 produces a vector of 1000 probabilities corresponding to the 1000 classes in the ImageNet dataset. The input image is assigned the class with the maximum probability.

Batch Normalization. Neural networks are often trained on small batches of input, sampled from a larger dataset. However, the distribution of values in the input batch varies across batches. This variation is referred to as 'covariate shift'.

Changes in distribution of input data can affect the behavior of neural networks. A neural network changes the weights of each layer through the course of its training, which in turn changes its activations. The distribution of the output of each layer changes over the course of the training, forcing the next layer to continuously adapt to these changes. Covariate shift extends the time required to train intermediate layers of the network.

Batch normalization [8] is applied to the output of each weighted layer to normalize their activations, with mean 0 and unit variance. This stabilizes the distribution of the input to the next layer and accelerates the training.

However, restricting these activations to values between 1 and −1 can be detrimental to learning. Thus, batch normalization layers learn parameters γ and β to scale and shift the normalized activations.

Batch normalization can also improve the performance of the network. VGG16 with batch normalization has a Top-1 error rate of 26.63%, as compared to simple

Table 1 Composition of datasets

Dataset	ALL	ALL subjects	NORMAL	NORMAL subjects
Training	7272	47	3389	26
Preliminary	1219	13	648	15
Final	Unknown	9	Unknown	8

VGG16 which has a Top-1 error rate of 28.41%. Top-1 error rate measures the error in predicting the correct class for the input image.

Transfer Learning. Training a CNN with random initialization is difficult and time-consuming and requires a large dataset. Training a network initialized with weights obtained from pretraining the network on a large dataset can reduce the time and data required for further training. This technique of using a pretrained network as an initialization is known as transfer learning. Finetuning is a form of transfer learning which updates all the parameters of the model to adapt to the new dataset.

The VGG16 network, pretrained on the large ImageNet dataset, exhibits a strong ability to generalize to images outside the ImageNet dataset through transfer learning. Hence, we chose to fine tune a VGG16 network to classify malignant leukemic cells versus normal blood cells.

3.1 Data

The training and test datasets provided consist of microscopic images of individual cells of two classes: ALL (malignant) and NORMAL. The data in both categories are drawn from multiple subjects who are given separate IDs. Refer to Table 1 for composition of datasets.

3.2 Data Preprocessing

The individual microscopic images are three-channel images of size 450 × 450. The images have been preprocessed using stain normalization to remove variations in illumination. Data acquisition and preprocessing have been described further in detail in [9–13].

The data in the NORMAL class were augmented by applying horizontal and vertical flips alongside rotation by 90°, 180°, and 270° to equalize the number of images in both classes.

The architecture of VGG16 only accepts 224 × 224 × 3-channel input. The input microscopic images must be first downsampled before being fed to the network. Since the images are of size 450 × 450, they are center cropped to obtain images of size 448 × 448. Since the border of these images belongs to the background, the

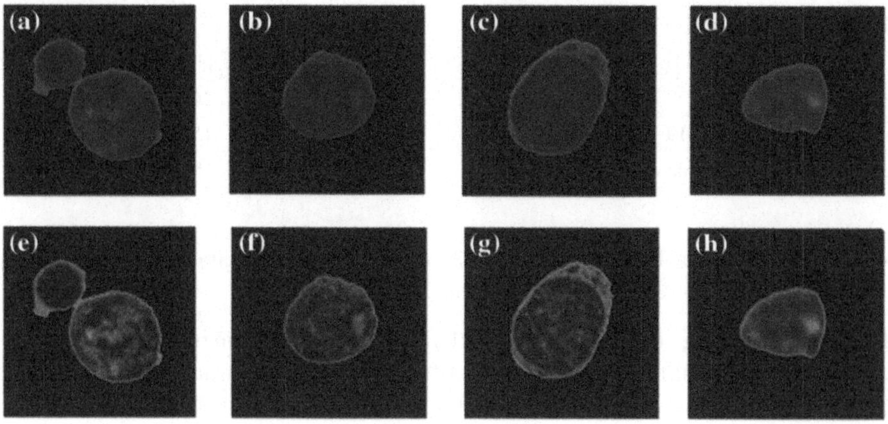

Fig. 3 **a–d** are samples from the preliminary test set. **e–h** are their corresponding contrast-enhanced versions. **a** and **d** are samples from the ALL class, while **b** and **c** are samples from the NORMAL class. After Stage 1 training, the network classifies **a** and **c** as ALL, and **b** and **d** as NORMAL

loss of information is minimal. The images are downsampled by a factor of 2 by a convolutional layer prepended to the VGG16 network.

Contrast-limited adaptive histogram equalization (CLAHE) was applied to all the images to enhance the contrast and finer details (refer to Fig. 3), before being fed to the network. The images are projected onto the YUV color space and CLAHE is performed exclusively on the Y channel. The image is then projected back to the RGB color space.

3.3 Finetuning

The network has the same architecture as the standard pretrained VGG16 network with batch normalization layers. A convolutional layer of three kernels of size 2×2 and stride 2, with ReLU activation, was prepended to the network to down sample the input images of size 448×448. The output of this layer has three channels of size 224×224 which can be fed to the original VGG16 network. This layer provides the advantage of learning the downsampling weights through training.

The final softmax layer of the network was reshaped to have only two outputs corresponding to each of the classes in the input data, NORMAL (0) and ALL (1) (refer to Fig. 2).

The training was carried out in stages. In Stage 1, the network was re-trained on the training data alone, while the preliminary test dataset was used for validation. The model was further finetuned for better performance on the validation set in Stage 2.

4 Observations

The training dataset was divided into batches of size 10, with 5 from each class. These batches were then fed to the network for training. The total number of batches came to 1455, with a dataset size of 14,550. The images in each batch were also subjected to horizontal and vertical flips, and rotation by 90°, 180°, and 270°, with a probability of 0.5 for each transformation.

4.1 *Stage 1 Training*

Cross-entropy Loss. Cross-entropy loss measures the performance of a classification model that outputs a probability value between 0 and 1 for each class. The target for the model is a one-hot encoded vector of labels, that is, a vector of labels consisting of 0s and a single 1 corresponding to the actual class of the input. The loss penalizes divergence of the predicted probability for the class from its target label. For example, a predicted probability of 0.1 for a class where the target label is 1 results in a large loss value.

$$\text{Cross Entropy Loss}\,(p, y) = -\Sigma_i y_i \log(p_i)$$
$$\text{for}\, i = 1, \ldots, K$$

where p is a vector of probabilities corresponding to K classes and y is a one-hot encoded vector of labels. The loss is average over each batch.

The network was trained using cross-entropy loss across the two classes. The loss was optimized using stochastic gradient descent with momentum = 0.9. The learning rate was set at 0.01 and halved every two epochs till the tenth epoch, and then halved every ten epochs. However, the best performance on the validation set was achieved within the first 10–15 epochs.

As can be observed from Fig. 4, applying CLAHE enhances the loss optimization of the network. Furthermore, we were able to achieve better performance on the validation set in applying CLAHE, as seen in Fig. 5.

4.2 *Stage 2 Training*

The model with the best performance on the validation set (weighted F1 score = 0.848966) was further finetuned for better performance on the final test dataset. The network was finetuned on a combination of the training and validation datasets used in Stage 1. Methods to finetune the performance included L2 regularization with regularizing coefficient $\lambda = 0.001$ and using a combination of cross-entropy and triplet loss.

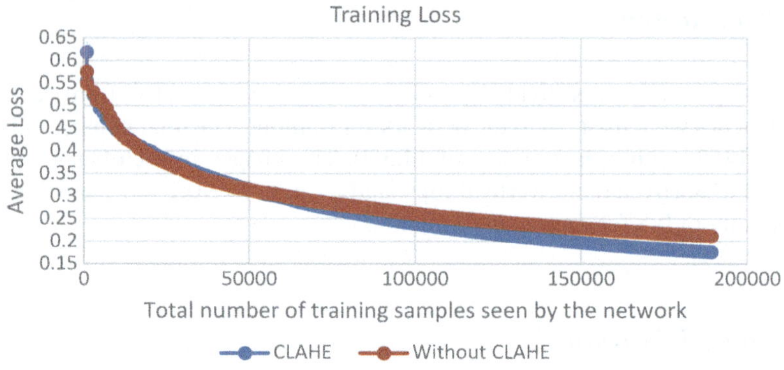

Fig. 4 Average training loss versus total number of training samples seen by the network, for (i) input with CLAHE applied and (ii) input without CLAHE applied. These training samples are not unique, as all the samples in a dataset are used once in every epoch. CLAHE parameters: clip limit = 2.0, grid size = 8 × 8

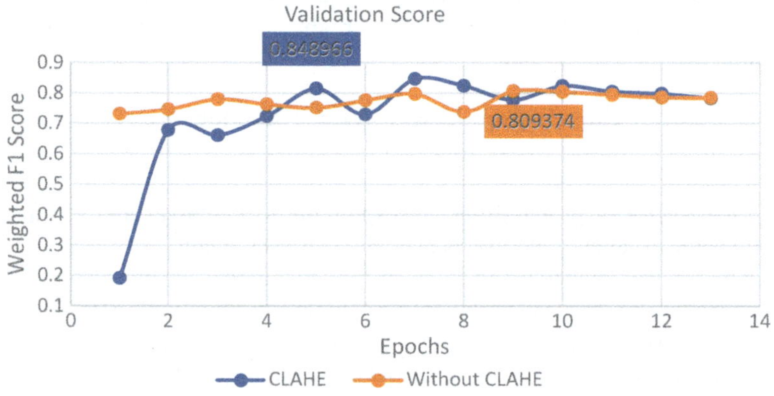

Fig. 5 Weighted F1 score for validation set versus epochs run for (i) input with CLAHE applied and (ii) input without CLAHE applied. Best scores are indicated by labeling the corresponding data point

Triplet Loss. Triplet loss measures the relative similarity within a triplet of samples. A triplet consists of a baseline sample (anchor, a), a positive sample (p), and a negative sample (n). The loss value magnifies as the similarity between a and p decreases or as the similarity between a and n increases. Similarity is most often measured in terms of their Euclidean distance.

$$L(a, p, n) = \max\{d(a_i, p_i) - d(a_i, n_i) + \text{margin}, 0\}$$
$$\text{for } i = 1, \ldots, K$$

where $d(x, y) = \|x - y\|_2$ is the Euclidean distance between x and y and K is the number of triplets in a batch. Training the network using triplet loss ensures that the features for the anchor and positive sample generated by the network are close together, while the features for the negative samples are separated from those of the anchor and positive sample by at least the margin value. The trained network generates features that can be easily clustered into classes, separated by the margin value.

A finetuning method that was attempted was to train the model using a combination of triplet loss and cross-entropy loss. The triplet loss was calculated over a batch of ten triplets from the batch of ten feature vectors computed by the network (before applying the softmax function). For each feature vector used as anchor, the feature vector of a sample of the same class, which is at the greatest Euclidean distance from the anchor, was chosen as the positive example. The feature vector of a sample of the other class with the least Euclidean distance from the anchor was chosen as the negative example.

Although L2 regularization optimizes the loss better than the other methods (refer Fig. 6), the performance on the preliminary test dataset is best when the network is trained on the combined dataset (refer Fig. 7).

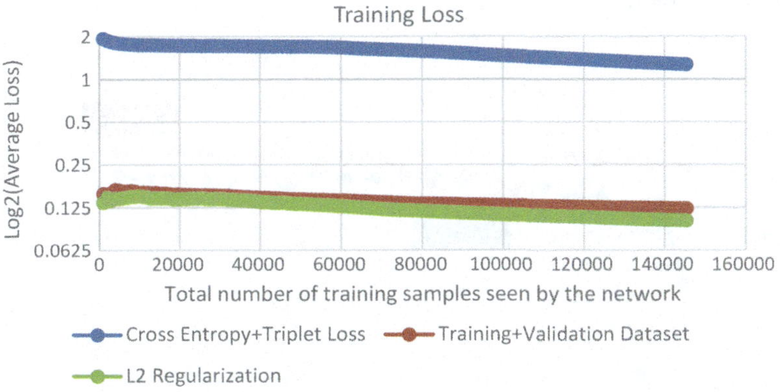

Fig. 6 Average training loss versus total number of training samples seen by the network, for finetuned model using (i) simple cross-entropy loss (training + validation dataset), (ii) cross-entropy loss with L2 regularization ($\lambda = 0.001$), and (iii) combined cross-entropy + triplet loss. These training samples are not unique, as all the samples in a dataset are used once in every epoch. The network was finetuned on a combination of the training and validation datasets used in Stage 1

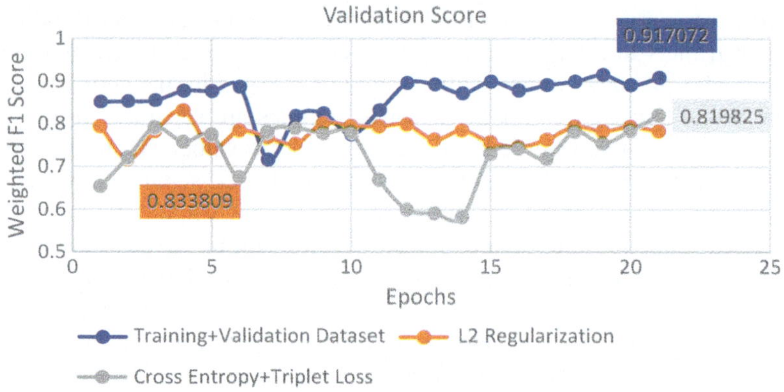

Fig. 7 Weighted F1 score for validation set versus epochs run, for finetuned model using (i) simple cross-entropy loss (training + validation dataset), (ii) cross-entropy loss with L2 regularization ($\lambda = 0.001$), and (iii) combined cross-entropy + triplet loss. Best scores are indicated by labeling the corresponding data point. The network was finetuned on a combination of the training and validation datasets used in Stage 1

5 Results

See Fig. 8 and Table 2.

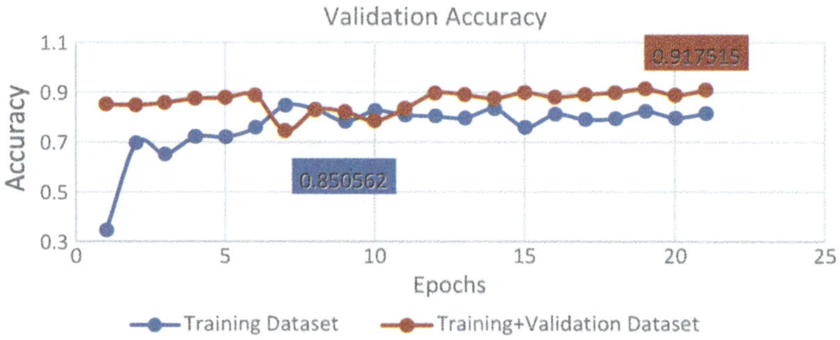

Fig. 8 Accuracy for validation set versus epochs run, for finetuned model using cross-entropy loss on (i) training dataset and (ii) combined training + validation dataset. Greatest accuracy for each method is indicated by labeling the corresponding data point

Table 2 Scores for test datasets

Dataset	Weighted precision	Weighted recall	Weighted-F1 score
Preliminary	0.917085	0.917515	0.917072
Final	Unknown	Unknown	0.8079664712

6 Conclusions

The problem of classifying malignant leukemic blasts versus normal cells can be addressed by finetuning a VGG16 network with batch normalization, pretrained on the 1000-class ImageNet dataset. Applying CLAHE to the input images before feeding them to the network for training helps improve the performance of the network. Further finetuning using simple cross-entropy loss on a combined training + validation dataset improves the performance of the model, as opposed to a finetuning using triplet and cross-entropy or cross-entropy loss with L2 regularization.

However, the VGG16 network has a few drawbacks. Training the network is a time-consuming process, as the network is deep and has a large number of parameters. The model weights are large and require large amounts of memory space for storage (~0.5 GB). This inhibits easy deployment. One can opt for a simpler, lighter model such as SqueezeNet [14] or DenseNet to further reduce the space and time complexity in comparison to VGG16. Adopting a smaller network architecture may help resolve the issue.

References

1. Krishna Kanth, B.B.M.: A fuzzy-neural approach for blood cancer classification. Int. J. Sci. Res. **2**(11) (2013). ISSN: 2277-8179
2. Adjouadi, M., Ayala, M., Cabrerizo, M., Zong, N., Lizarraga G., Rossman, M.: Classification of blood cancer blood samples using neural networks. Ann. Biomed. Eng. **38**(4), 1473–1482 (2010)
3. Krishna Kanth, B.B.M., Kulkarni, U.V., Giridhar, B.G.V.: Gene expression based acute blood cancer cancer classification-a neuro fuzzy approach. Int. J. Biometr. Bioinf. (IJBB) **4**(4)
4. Amin, M.M., Kermani, S., Talebi, A., Oghli, M.G.: Recognition of acute lymphoblastic blood cancer cells in microscopic images using K-means clustering and support vector machine classifier. J. Med. Signals Sens. **5**(1) (2015)
5. Simonyan, K., Zisserman, A.: Very deep convolutional networks for large-scale image recognition. CoRR (2014). arXiv:1409.1556
6. ImageNet Large Scale Visual Recognition Challenge. http://www.image-net.org/challenges/LSVRC/
7. ImageNet. http://image-net.org/
8. Ioffe, S., Szegedy, C.: Batch normalization: accelerating deep network training by reducing internal covariate shift. In: Bach, F., Blei, D. (eds.) Proceedings of the 32nd International Conference on International Conference on Machine Learning (ICML'15), vol. 37. pp. 448–456 (2015). JMLR.org
9. Gupta, A., Duggal, R., Gupta, R., Kumar, L., Thakkar, N., Satpathy, D.: GCTI-SN: geometry-inspired chemical and tissue invariant stain normalization of microscopic medical images. Under review
10. Gupta, R., Mallick, P., Duggal, R., Gupta, A., Sharma, O.: Stain color normalization and segmentation of plasma cells in microscopic images as a prelude to development of computer assisted automated disease diagnostic tool in multiple Myeloma. In: 16th International Myeloma Workshop (IMW), India, March 2017
11. Duggal, R., Gupta, A., Gupta, R., Wadhwa, M., Ahuja, C.: Overlapping cell nuclei segmentation in microscopic images using deep belief networks. In: Indian Conference on Computer Vision, Graphics and Image Processing (ICVGIP), India, December 2016

12. Duggal, R., Gupta, A., Gupta, A.: Segmentation of overlapping/touching white blood cell nuclei using artificial neural networks. CME Series on Hemato-Oncopathology, All India Institute of Medical Sciences (AIIMS), New Delhi, India, July 2016
13. Duggal, R., Gupta, A., Gupta, R., Mallick, P.: SD-layer: stain deconvolutional layer for CNNs in medical microscopic imaging. In: Descoteaux, M., Maier-Hein, L., Franz, A., Jannin, P., Collins, D., Duchesne, S. (eds.) Medical Image Computing and Computer-Assisted Intervention, MICCAI 2017. Lecture Notes in Computer Science, Part III, LNCS 10435, pp. 435–443. Springer, Cham. https://doi.org/10.1007/978-3-319-66179-7_50
14. Iandola, F.N., et al.: SqueezeNet: AlexNet-level accuracy with 50x fewer parameters and <1 MB model size. CoRR (2017). arXiv:1602.07360

Classification of Leukemic B-Lymphoblast Cells from Blood Smear Microscopic Images with an Attention-Based Deep Learning Method and Advanced Augmentation Techniques

Christian Marzahl, Marc Aubreville, Jörn Voigt and Andreas Maier

Abstract Acute Lymphoblastic Leukemia (ALL) is a blood cell cancer type characterized by an increased number of immature lymphocytes. It is one of the leading cancer inflicted causes of death among children and affected around 876.000 people globally in 2015. In this work, we describe methods used for the "Classification of Normal versus Malignant Cells in B-ALL White Blood Cancer Microscopic Images" ISBI challenge. Due to the morphological similarity between malignant and normal cells, the classification of these cell types is a very challenging task, even for human experts. Deep learning using Convolutional Neural Networks (CNN) provides state-of-the-art techniques for image classification, even with limited annotation data, based on techniques like transfer learning and data augmentation. Our solution to tackle this classification problem is based upon advanced augmentation techniques to counter overfitting the small dataset and transfer learning with adaptive learning rates. Additionally, we incorporated a basic attention mechanism based on a region proposal subnetwork to boost our results for this competition. The ResNet 18 network with an additional regression head achieved a weighted F1 score of 0.8284 on the final test set and 0.8746 on the preliminary test set.

Keywords Deep learning · Acute Lymphoblastic Leukemia · Attention modeling

C. Marzahl · M. Aubreville · A. Maier
Pattern Recognition Lab, Computer Science, Friedrich-Alexander-Universität Erlangen-Nürnberg, Erlangen, Germany

C. Marzahl (✉) · J. Voigt
Research & Development Projects, EUROIMMUN Medizinische Labordiagnostika AG, Lübeck, Germany
e-mail: c.marzahl@euroimmun.de

A. Gupta and R. Gupta (eds.), *ISBI 2019 C-NMC Challenge: Classification in Cancer Cell Imaging*, Lecture Notes in Bioengineering,
https://doi.org/10.1007/978-981-15-0798-4_2

1 Introduction

Acute Lymphoblastic Leukemia (ALL) is a blood cell cancer type characterized by developing an increase in the number of immature lymphocytes. With a global incidence rate of 876,000 people and a mortality rate of 110,500 people (both in 2015 [17, 18]), it is one of the leading cancer inflicted causes of death among children. However, following early detection and with sufficient medical care, ALL reaches an overall cure rate of 80% [10]. Consequently, it is important to attain early and accurate diagnosis. Classification of ALL and normal cells is a challenging task due to their visual similarity (see Fig. 1a). To address this there have been some attempts to propose automated approaches to address similar tasks, like Vogado et al. [16], who used a pre-trained VGG-16 for feature extraction and an ensemble of non-deep learning-based classifiers on the extracted features. Shafique et al. [14] utilized a deep learning approach based on AlexNet and transfer learning with additional fine-tuning of the feature extractor. Duggal et al. [5] used a special stain deconvolutional layer to improve performance on two standard CNN architectures for white blood cells cancer classification.

In this paper, we propose a novel deep learning-based pipeline comprising an ensemble of five models with a dedicated preprocessing and augmentation stage, each model trained leaving out onefold of the available training set. As a novel approach, in this work, we customize the standard training pipeline with the following adjustments:

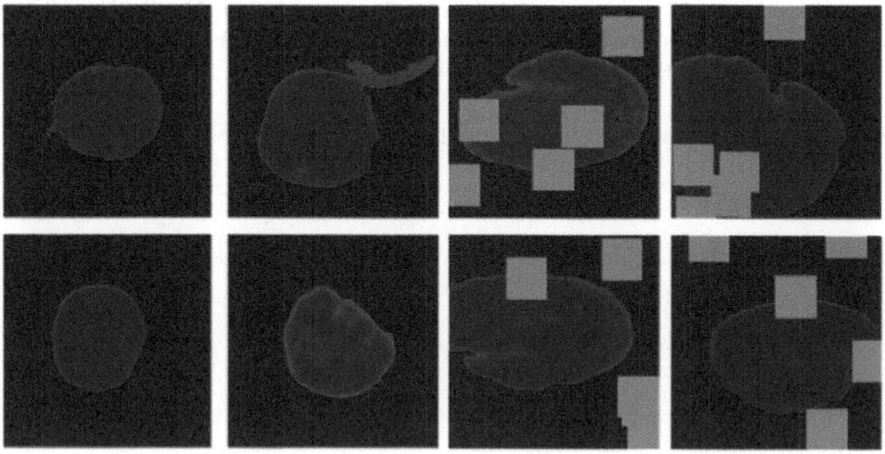

(a) data set (b) Augmented images

Fig. 1 **a** Example images from the challenge dataset. Top row: ALL cells. Bottom row: normal cells. **b** Visualization of all (except mixup) applied augmentation techniques

- We utilize model attention using a dedicated regression head in a multitask learning scenario.
- We perform model selection based on the MCC score [1, 9].
- We make use of an advanced data augmentation technique.

2 Material

The dataset was provided as part of the ISBI White Blood Cell Cancer Challenge and consists of single-cell images segmented from bone marrow aspirate slide images with a size of 2560 × 1920 pixels, which were dyed using Jenner-Giemsa stain. Each cell is roughly of size 300 × 300 pixels. The slide images were stain normalized [7] before the segmentation of single lymphoblasts. The resulting training data for this challenge consist of 10,661 white blood cell images, divided into two classes: Acute Lymphocytic Leukemia (ALL) containing 7,272 examples and normal (hem) containing 3,389 examples. The images belong to 76 individual subjects and 47 ALL subjects compared to 29 healthy (hem) subjects. The number of examples per patient is highly imbalanced. The mean number of images per patient in the ALL class is 155 ($\min = 9$, $\max = 757$) and 130 ($\min = 9$, $\max = 405$) in the normal class. Each image contains only one cell which is padded with black pixels to reach the size of 450 by 450 pixels (Fig. 1a).

The preliminary test set, as provided by the competition, includes 1219 additional ALL images from 13 subjects and 648 images from 15 healthy subjects. In this preliminary test set, the mean number of images per patient is 93 ($\min = 7$, $\max = 262$) in the ALL class and 43 ($\min = 5$, $\max = 162$) in the normal class. The final test set contains 2586 images with an unknown patient and class affiliation.

3 Methods

In this paper, we propose a deep learning-based pipeline utilizing a dedicated preprocessing scheme with normalization and two augmentation methods. For training, we split the data into fivefold on subject level and use a ResNet18 network [8] for classification and an additional regression head for bounding box prediction. During inference, the models are ensembled using a majority vote on the classification results.

The code for all experiments is available online.[1]

[1] https://github.com/ChristianMarzahl/ISBI2019_WhiteBloodCancer.

3.1 Data Normalization

Input normalization is known to speed up convergence of deep neuronal networks. One standard technique for this is subtraction of the mean and division by the variance of the training mini-batch. For the given task, we propose to use this method only for the foreground (i.e., cell) pixels and the background pixels remained unaltered.

3.2 Data Augmentation

Due to the limited training data, which consists of around 8000 images per fold, we made extensive use of data augmentation to increase the effective size of the training set. We used standard techniques for microscopy images such as

1. Horizontal and vertical flip,
2. Rotation up to 90°,
3. Scaling of the image,
4. Intensity augmentation (e.g., contrast enhancement, constant intensity offsets), and
5. Tilting the image in each direction (left, right, top, bottom) with a positive and negative magnitude.

Additionally, we made use of some recently developed augmentation techniques like mixup [19] and cutout [3] (see Fig. 1b).

3.3 Data Split

Initially, the data were split into threefold. To increase the training data per fold, we created a fivefold split, complying with two conditions: each fold has to have approximately the same ratio of normal cells to ALL cells as the original data and images pertaining to the same subject may not be split across folds. We achieved this by splitting the subjects into two lists, one for normal and one for ALL and then sorting them by the number of images per subject. The second step was to assign the subjects to folds by putting the subject with the fewest images in the first fold, the subject next on the list (sorted low to high) in the second fold, and so on. After the fifth fold, the assigning system was reversed to keep the numbers balanced (see Table 1).

3.4 Predicting the Bounding Box

According to Bain [2], cell size is one criterion that can be used to differentiate normal from ALL cells. To take advantage of this knowledge, we challenged the

Table 1 Fivefold data split of the training data provided by the authors of the challenge. Note that the original split included only threefold

Fold	Normal	ALL
0	449	1218
1	571	1225
2	629	1192
3	654	1951
4	1086	1686
Total	3389	7272

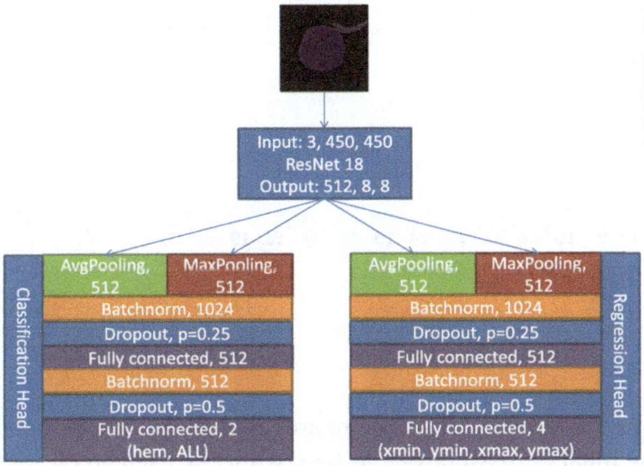

(a) Network overview

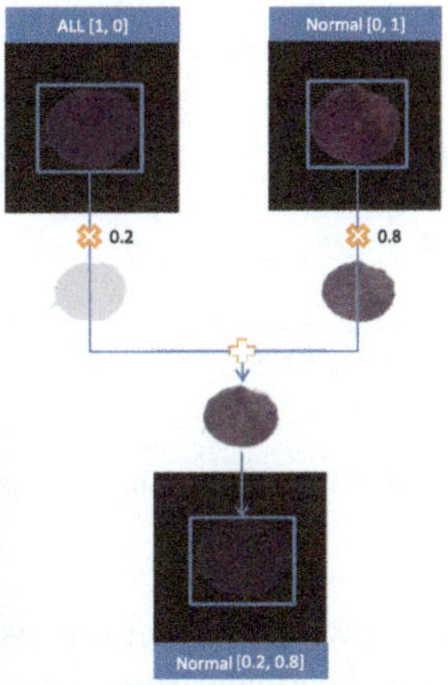

(b) Mixup augmentation technique

Fig. 2 Implementation details of the network topology. A ResNet 18 [8] base network was extended with two heads, one for classification and another for regression of bounding boxes. Right: Mixup [19] was used as additional augmentation technique

deep neuronal network to predict both the classification result and a bounding box for the cell. By predicting the bounding box, we incorporated an attention mechanism into the network architecture. Additionally, we adopted the mixup technique [19] to align both cells with the bounding box (see Fig. 2b).

3.5 *Neuronal Network Model Architecture*

Due to the limited number of examples, we used a compact ResNet18 architecture pre-trained on ImageNet [13] with two custom heads: one for classification and one regression head for bounding box prediction (Fig. 2a).

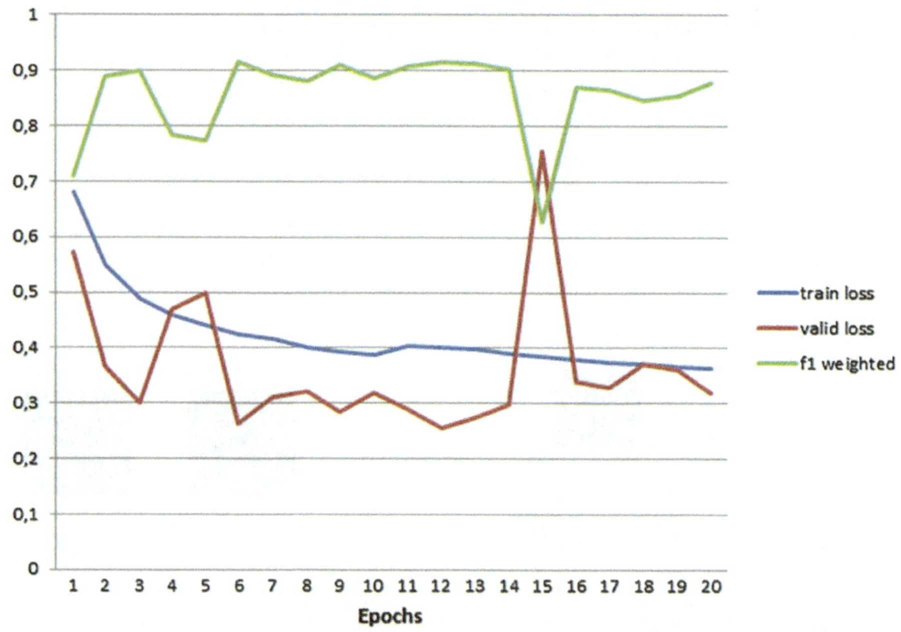

Fig. 3 Loss and weighted F1 score evolution for the first fold

Loss Two loss functions were combined to train the neuronal network: the classification head was trained using binary cross-entropy as loss, while we used an L1 loss for the bounding box regression. Both components were added up, while the binary cross-entropy loss was scaled according to the mixup factor of the batch samples.

Training The network was trained using the Adam optimizer with a maximum learning rate of 0.01 and a weight decay value of 0.001. For each batch, the learning rate was set according to the cyclical learning rate technique [15]. For the first ten epochs only, the classification and regression head were trained, while the weights of ResNet18 were frozen. After the initial ten epochs, the whole network was optimized for another ten epochs (see Fig. 3). We employ the MCC score [1] to select the model with highest score on the validation set. This process is repeated for each fold, resulting in a total number of five models.

Inference During inference, we employ Test-Time Augmentation (TTA). For this, each image is classified four times per model, using all abovementioned augmentation techniques. Final classification is retrieved by averaging and thresholding the outputs. Five models process the images in this manner; subsequently, a majority vote yields the final result.

4 Results

On the preliminary test set, we find that our approach reaches a weighted F1 score of 0.874 and on the final test set of 0.8284. In comparison to the baseline setup with a vanilla ResNet18 implementation (0.859), we see the advantage of the chosen approach (see Table 2 for a detailed lineup).

The resulting precision, recall, and F1-Score on the preliminary test set for each class are presented in Table 3. We calculated these values for the case when the assignment between image and subject being unknown (evaluation per image) and when the assignment is known (evaluation per subject). For the latter, the classification of images pertaining to the same subject was adjusted according to the majority of votes, i.e., if the majority of images belonging to one subject were classified as ALL, the classification of the remaining images was changed from normal to ALL. This postprocessing step increased the F1-Score from 0.876 to 0.926.

We also computed the box–whisker plots for each class visualized in Fig. 4a and the accuracy per subject as a spider chart shown in Fig. 4b. See Fig. 5 for images from normal subjects where the network prediction was incorrect.

Table 2 Ablation study as per results on the preliminary test set for the proposed architecture. All results produced by ensemble of five models

Refinement	Weighted F1-Score
ResNet18	0.859
+ cell normalization	0.862
+ Cutout [3]	0.864
+ Attention (bounding box regression)	0.869
+ MixUp [19]	0.871
+ TTA	0.874

Table 3 Precision, recall, and F1-Score for each class with and without subject affiliation

Class	Patient assignment unknown			Patient assignment known		
	Precision	Recall	Weighted F1	Precision	Recall	Weighted F1
ALL	0.884	0.931	0.907	0.901	1	0.948
Normal	0.857	0.771	0.812	1	0.794	0.885
Average	0.875	0.876	0.874	0.935	0.928	0.926

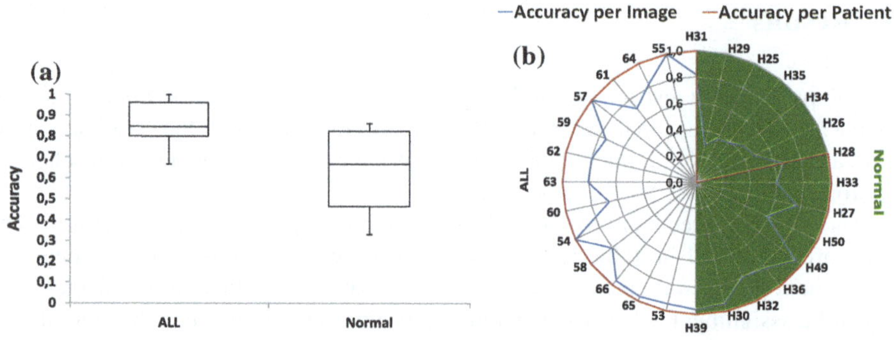

Fig. 4 Evaluation of the proposed approach on the preliminary test set. The left panel shows the distribution of accuracy in both groups. The right panel shows individual results, where all subjects with ALL diagnosis are depicted on the left and all subjects with negative result for ALL are depicted on the right

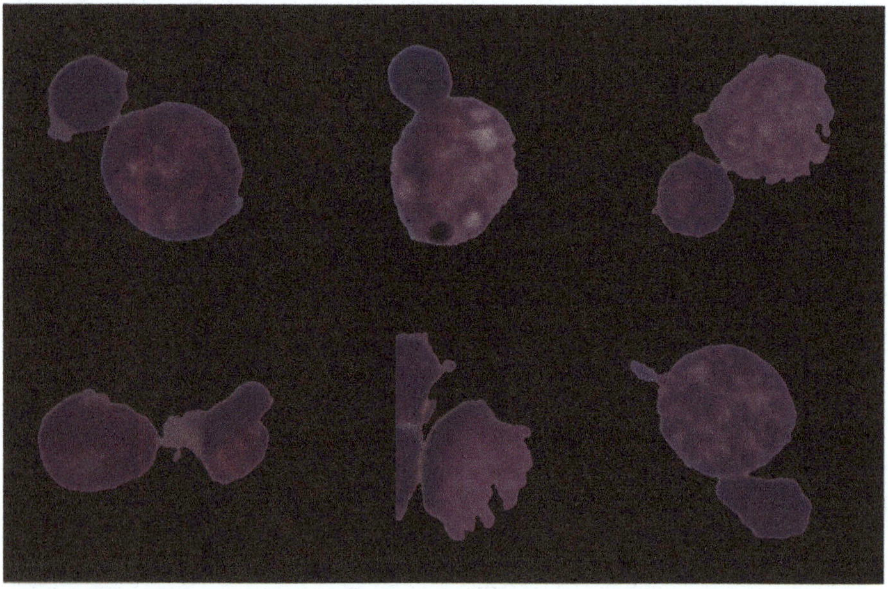

Fig. 5 Six exemplary images taken from the preliminary test set, showing cropping artifacts and multiple cells per image

5 Discussion

The images used for classification in the challenge dataset partially included severe cropping artifacts (see Fig. 5) caused by the segmentation [4, 6] in preprocessing. These images constituted an especially high proportion of all misclassified images. We thus hypothesize that the performance of the presented approach would significantly benefit from either perfect segmentation in the preprocessing or even from the absence of prior cropping in general. Deep learning algorithms typically benefit from incorporating contextual knowledge provided by the environment of the detected or classified object. Besides preventing the occurrence of cropping artifacts, this would also allow the network to utilize meta-information such as cellular density. Furthermore, this would enable the use of state-of-the-art deep learning object detection methods [11, 12] for this task.

References

1. Andersen, C.A.F., Nielsen, H., Baldi, P., et al.: Assessing the accuracy of prediction algorithms for classification: an overview. Bioinformatics **16**(5), 412–424 (2000). https://doi.org/10.1093/bioinformatics/16.5.412.
2. Bain, B.J.: Blood Cells: A Practical Guide. Wiley (2014)
3. DeVries, T., Taylor, G.W.: Improved regularization of convolutional neural networks with cutout (2017). arXiv:1708.04552
4. Duggal, R., Gupta, A., Gupta, R.: Segmentation of overlapping/touching white blood cell nuclei using artificial neural networks. In: CME Series on Hemato-Oncopathology. AIIMS (2016)
5. Duggal, R., Gupta, A., Gupta, R., et al.: SD-layer: stain deconvolutional layer for CNNs in medical microscopic imaging. In: Descoteaux, M., Maier-Hein, L., Franz, A., et al. (eds.) Medical Image Computing and Computer Assisted Intervention MICCAI 2017, pp. 435–443. Springer International Publishing, Cham (2017)
6. Duggal, R., Gupta, A., Gupta, R., et al.: Overlapping cell nuclei segmentation in microscopic images using deep belief networks. In: Proceedings of the Tenth Indian Conference on Computer Vision, Graphics and Image Processing, p. 82. ACM (2016)
7. Gupta, R., Mallick, P., Duggal, R., et al.: Stain color normalization and segmentation of plasma cells in microscopic images as a prelude to development of computer assisted automated disease diagnostic tool in multiple myeloma. Clin. Lymphoma Myeloma Leukemia **17**(1), e99 (2017)
8. He, K., Zhang, X., Ren, S., et al.: Deep residual learning for image recognition. In: 2016 IEEE Conference on Computer Vision and Pattern Recognition (CVPR), pp. 770–778. IEEE (2016)
9. Matthews, B.W.: Comparison of the predicted and observed secondary structure of T4 phage lysozyme. Biochimica et Biophysica Acta (BBA)-Protein Struct. **405**(2), 442–451 (1975)
10. Pui, C.H., Evans, W.E.: Treatment of acute lymphoblastic leukemia. New Engl. J. Med. **354**(2), 166–178 (2006)
11. Redmon, J., Divvala, S., Girshick, R., et al.: You only look once: unified, real-time object detection. In: Proceedings of the IEEE Conference on Computer Vision and Pattern Recognition, pp. 779–788 (2016)
12. Ren, S., He, K., Girshick, R., et al.: Faster R-CNN: towards real-time object detection with region proposal networks. In: Advances in Neural Information Processing Systems, pp. 91–99 (2015)
13. Russakovsky, O., Deng, J., Su, H., et al.: Imagenet large scale visual recognition challenge. Int. J. Comput. Vis. **115**(3), 211–252 (2015)

14. Shafique, S., Tehsin, S.: Acute lymphoblastic leukemia detection and classification of its subtypes using pretrained deep convolutional neural networks. Technol. Cancer Res. Treat. **17**, 1533033818802789 (2018)
15. Smith, L.N.: Cyclical learning rates for training neural networks. In: 2017 IEEE Winter Conference on Applications of Computer Vision (WACV), pp. 464–472. IEEE (2017)
16. Vogado, L.H.S., Veras, R.D.M.S., Andrade, A.R., et al.: Diagnosing leukemia in blood smear images using an ensemble of classifiers and pre-trained convolutional neural networks. In: 2017 30th SIBGRAPI Conference on Graphics, Patterns and Images (SIBGRAPI), pp. 367–373. IEEE (2017)
17. Vos, T., Allen, C., Arora, M., et al.: Global, regional, and national incidence, prevalence, and years lived with disability for 310 diseases and injuries, 1990–2015: a systematic analysis for the Global Burden of Disease Study 2015. The Lancet **388**(10053), 1545–1602 (2016)
18. Wang, H., Naghavi, M., Allen, C., et al.: Global, regional, and national life expectancy, all-cause mortality, and cause-specific mortality for 249 causes of death, 1980–2015: a systematic analysis for the global burden of disease study 2015. The Lancet **388**(10053), 1459–1544 (2016)
19. Zhang, H., Cisse, M., Dauphin, Y.N., et al.: mixup: Beyond empirical risk minimization (2017). arXiv:1710.09412

Classification of Normal and Leukemic Blast Cells in B-ALL Cancer Using a Combination of Convolutional and Recurrent Neural Networks

Salman Shah, Wajahat Nawaz, Bushra Jalil and Hassan Aqeel Khan

Abstract Acute Lymphocytic or Lymphoblastic Leukemia (ALL) is a virulent form of blood cancer that affects white blood cells and the bone-marrow–spongy tissue. At the start of ALL, immature white blood cells proliferate and replace healthy cells in the bone marrow. ALL progresses quickly and can be fatal within a few months if not treated. Computer assisted diagnosis and prognosis of ALL, therefore, has the potential to save many lives but requires high accuracy classification of malignant cells which is challenging due to the visual similarity between normal and malignant cells. In this work, we employ a custom-built deep learning model for the classification of immature lymphoblasts and normal cells. Our model is an ensemble of convolutional and recurrent neural networks. It also exploits the spectral features of the cells by using discrete cosine transform in conjunction with an RNN. The proposed classifier has been validated using multiple experiments. Our approach is able to achieve substantial performance gains when compared to, conventional, stand-alone CNN- and RNN-based methods. The highest accuracy achieved by our model is 86.6%.

Keywords Convolutional neural networks · Recurrent neural networks · LSTM · DCT · Ensemble models · Fine-tuning · Acute Lymphocytic or Lymphoblastic Leukemia

---

S. Shah (✉) · W. Nawaz · H. A. Khan
National University of Science and Technology, Islamabad, Pakistan
e-mail: sshah.msee16seecs@seecs.edu.pk

W. Nawaz
e-mail: wnawaz@seecs.edu.pk

H. A. Khan
e-mail: hassan.aqeel@seecs.edu.pk

B. Jalil
Istituto di Scienza e Tecnologie delĺInformazione, "Alessandro Faedo"
Area della Ricerca CNR di Pisa, Pisa, Italy
e-mail: bushra.jalil@isti.cnr.it

A. Gupta and R. Gupta (eds.), *ISBI 2019 C-NMC Challenge: Classification in Cancer Cell Imaging*, Lecture Notes in Bioengineering,
https://doi.org/10.1007/978-981-15-0798-4_3

1 Introduction

Acute Lymphoblastic Leukemia (ALL) is a type of blood cancer that causes rapid production of abnormal white blood cells which eventually results in an immune system disorder. These abnormal cells can also migrate to different organs of the body, causing them to malfunction. ALL can also block the generation of red blood cells (RBC) and platelets. According to the American Cancer Society, among children with ALL, around 80–85% have B-cell ALL (B-ALL for short) which starts in B cells. Current approaches for ALL diagnosis include complete blood cell counts (via flow cytometry), bone marrow aspiration, and microscopic examination of the blood smear. Unfortunately, these techniques require either trained medical professionals or expensive hardware. Consequently, diagnostic services are still not accessible in many regions of the developing world. The rapid progression of this disease means that survival outlook for the majority of patients in underserved areas is bleak since their cancer would already be at the advanced stages by the time they reach a doctor. These limitations motivate the need for simple, low-cost, and automated diagnostic solutions. Recent improvements in computer vision algorithms and demonstration of almost human-level performance on a number of complex image analysis tasks make them an appealing option for a computer aided diagnostic solution for this problem. In this work, we investigate novel deep learning models that can classify "leukemic" B-lymphoblast cells and "normal" B-lymphoid precursors using microscopic images of blood smears with high accuracy.

The primary challenge facing an image-based diagnostic system is the morphological similarity between the normal and malignant cells. Due to the limited size of the training data, we have limited ourselves to fine-tuning of the existing CNN and RNN models [8, 9], however, instead of limiting ourselves to fine-tuning standalone models, we try various combinations of popular deep learning architectures. Two broad strategies are employed for combining different (fine-tuned) models. Our first strategy is to employ a joint *CNN-RNN based Feature Learner* followed by a neural network classifier. This approach employs DenseNet proposed by Gao Huang [9] for learning visual features that discriminate between the classes of cells. In parallel to the DenseNet block, an LSTM network is used for learning contextual dependencies. We refer to this model as LSTM-DENSE.

Our second strategy is to use *Ensemble*-based learning to combine LSTM-DENSE with a pretrained (AlexNet [11]) CNN architecture. Moreover, we add a third model to this ensemble. This model employs DCT features which have been shown to be quite discriminative for ALL cell classification [4, 10, 21]. Taking inspiration from [10], we pass these DCT features to an LSTM with the objective of learning contextual dependencies in the spectral domain.

This paper is organized as follows: A brief overview of related approaches in the existing literature is presented in Sect. 2. Section 3.1 describes the dataset and preprocessing techniques employed. The architectures employed for classification are discussed in Sect. 3.2. Section 4 presents the results of different architectures used. Conclusions are presented at the very end in Sect. 5.

2 Related Work

A large number of existing works on ALL classification and segmentation have employed handcrafted features. For example, a dual thresholding method was used for blast cell segmentation in [13]; ALL classification was performed using conventional machine learning techniques in [15]. The exceptional results demonstrated by deep learning have led to a resurgence of interest in neural networks. Consequently, a large number of recent works on cancer screening and diagnosis have employed deep learning based approaches. However, due to the limited size of training sets, most of these approaches have been confined to fine-tuning of the existing models. For example, an AlexNet [11]-based model was employed for the classification of breast cancer histology images in [14]; classification of cervical cells was performed by fine-tuning a CNN in [22]. A high accuracy breast cancer screening algorithm using mammograms was developed by fine-tuning the existing popular CNN architectures in [2]. The efficacy of fine-tuning on a number of medical imaging tasks was examined in [19]; authors demonstrated that fine-tuned CNNs are better or just similar to CNNs trained from scratch. In addition to fine-tuning of standalone models, a few authors have also employed ensembles of fine-tuned, deep models for medical image classification [12, 16] and segmentation [1] tasks. A combination of two parallel CNN models was employed for B-ALL classification in [10].

Approaches based on combinations of CNNs and RNNs have previously been employed in other domains. For example, sentiment analysis was done on short texts in [20]; CNN was employed to learn local dependencies whereas long-term dependencies were learnt using an RNN. In [18], low-level, translational invariant features are learnt via a CNN layer and then input to RNNs to learn higher order features for classification of 3D objects. In [23], RNN layers were introduced into a fully convolutional neural network (FCN) for the detection of human skin. Our strategy of using a joint CNN-RNN architecture is, therefore, one of the first approaches to use this type of architecture for a B-ALL classification problem.

3 Methodology

3.1 Dataset Description and Preprocessing

The dataset used in this work has been obtained from the B-ALL normal versus malignant cells classification challenge of ISBI 2019. This dataset contains labeled normal and malignant cells images. These cells have been segmented from raw microscopic images after stain normalization using the approach described in [3, 5–7]. There are a total of 10,661 training images from 76 subjects, out of which 7,272 images are taken from 47 patients of ALL and 3,389 are taken from 29 normal subjects having healthy normal cells. We evaluated a large number of distinct models and thus divided the training into three folds and employed cross validation to identify

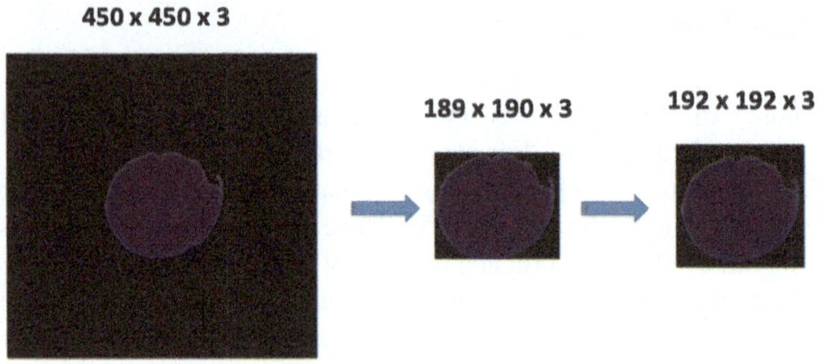

Fig. 1 Cropping contours and resizing operation

the best performing models and tweak their parameters. Our proposed network only accepts inputs of size 192 $\times$ 192 $\times$ 3 whereas the size of images from the dataset is 450 $\times$ 450 $\times$ 3. Since the majority of images contain redundant pixels outside of the actual cell region, instead of downsampling the whole image (and losing useful texture information), we use a crop contour based preprocessing method for extracting the useful portion of the image (contains only the regions containing cells portion). The dimension of the extracted cell might be less than the expected input dimension; to overcome this problem, the resizing operation is employed to obtain the desired input size by using zero padding. The complete cropping and resizing process is illustrated in Fig. 1. The original dataset is not balanced; data augmentation is employed to, somewhat, balance the training set and to reduce overfitting. Early on, only simple image rotation and horizontal and vertical flip operations were used for augmentation, however, we observed that by later addition, Gaussian blurring and shearing also had a positive impact on the training performance; consequently, these operations were also used for augmentation purposes.

3.2 Classification Architecture

Computer vision over the last few years has been dominated by data-driven approaches which are less restrictive than conventional approaches that rely on handcrafted approaches. However, large-scale data-driven models generally require a significant amount of labeled training data which is not available in most medical applications, due to the high cost associated with obtaining annotations from qualified physicians. We, therefore restrict ourselves to fine-tuning (or transfer learning) of the existing architectures, for the most part. The first approach we tried on this problem was simple fine-tuning of popular pretrained CNN models such as [9, 11, 17]. The performance of these standalone models was reasonable, however, we felt that more performance gains could be obtained by creating an ensemble of these models. Results demonstrate that this is indeed the case. The ensemble model performed well

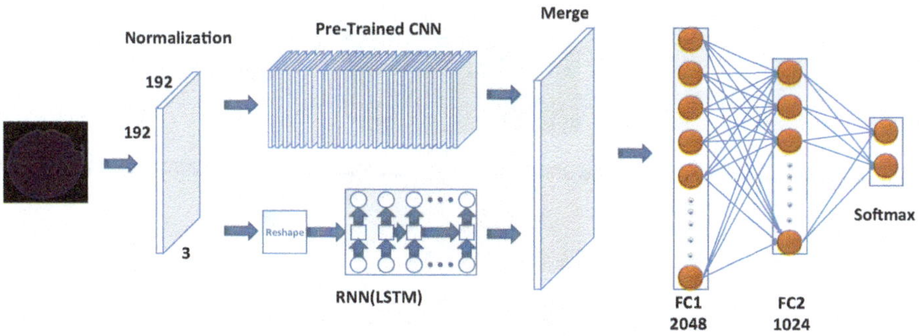

Fig. 2 LSTM-DENSE; this model combines a DenseNet CNN model with an LSTM

on the validation data but performance degraded on the test data on which accuracy saturated at around 76%. CNNs generally tend to be good at learning local dependencies; therefore, we hypothesized that the incorporation of more distant contextual dependencies, via a recurrent neural network, should result in further performance improvement. Consequently, we decided to use add an LSTM block to our model, which we refer to as the LSTM-DENSE architecture. This model is illustrated in Fig. 2; it consists of a CNN (DenseNet) and an LSTM and takes $192 \times 192 \times 3$ size images as input, feeds them to the LSTM and pretrained CNN models simultaneously. The LSTM layer accepts only 1D sequences, so the image is reshaped to a vector before being input to the LSTM. The outputs of both the models are merged using an averaging operation. In the end, two fully connected layers, followed by a Soft-max layer complete the network. The LSTM-DENSE model performed well on the dataset and achieved accuracy of 81.95% on the test data in Phase 2 of ISBI 2019 challenge. The accuracy of LSTM-DENSE is further improved by combining it with AlexNet [11], trained on the dataset separately. The ensemble model performed well on the test data, however, further performance gains may still be obtained by adding more models to our ensemble. A strong candidate for addition to our existing ensemble is a model that employs features based on the Discrete Cosine Transform (DCT). A CNN model preceded by a DCT layer has demonstrated excellent performance on the B-ALL classification task in [10]. We therefore, added a similar model to our ensemble. However (in contrast to [10]), we used an LSTM instead of a CNN after the DCT layer. Our final architecture is an ensemble of three models: (1) A PreTrained AlexNet model; (2) An LSTM-DENSE models, and (3) A hybrid DCT-LSTM model. This model is shown in Fig. 3. The final classification decision is made by averaging the values predicted by the three individual models in the ensemble. To the best of our knowledge, this is the first application of DCT-based RNN in a medical imaging application. Results demonstrate that the addition of the DCT-LSTM model delivers substantial performance gains.

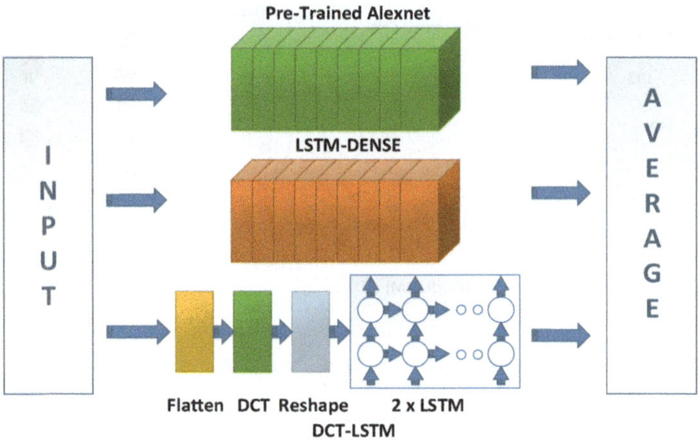

Fig. 3 The final model is a combination of a pretrained CNN (AlexNet), a hybrid CNN-RNN (LSTM-DENSE), and a sequential DCT-LSTM model

4 Results

During our initial experiments, we explored the fine-tuning of various popular CNN architectures. The dataset was originally divided into three folders based on subject level variation, so we used 3-fold cross validation. Initially, the dataset was used without data preprocessing, and standard resize operation was used since these architectures accept images of size $192 \times 192 \times 3$. The initial performance of the fine-tuned models was not great due to class imbalance. Consequently, the dataset was balanced using standard image transformation techniques (such as rotation and flipping). This resolved the biasing problem. Resizing based on cropping contours was also applied according to the method described in Sect. 3.1. Table 1 shows the performance of the fine-tuned models after class balancing, preprocessing, and data augmentation. The F1-scores for detection of normal and ALL cells ($F1_{hem}$ and $F1_{all}$) are also presented, in addition to the accuracy. The best performing stand-alone CNN model was AlexNet, which is somewhat surprising since in general, more recent models tend to be better on most tasks. One possible reason for this could be that the limited size of training data makes AlexNet more suitable for this task than newer but deeper architectures. Superior performance to other fine-tuned models is the main reason why we have used AlexNet in our final ensemble model (Fig. 3). We refer to the fine-tuning of stand-alone CNN models as **Phase 1** of our training process. In the subsequent phase (**Phase 2**), we trained the LSTM-DENSE model (Fig. 2); the training and validation curves for Phase 2 are plotted in Fig. 4. This model achieved a test accuracy of 81.95%. This is a significant improvement over the 76% test accuracy obtained for the AlexNet model in Phase 1.

In **Phase 3**, the AlexNet and LSTM-DENSE models are combined. This yields an accuracy of 83.81% on the test set on the second phase of the challenge.

Table 1 Performance comparison of different CNN models (Phase 1)

Model name	Fold 2			Fold 1			Fold 0		
	Acc	$F1_{hem}$	$F1_{all}$	Acc	$F1_{hem}$	$F1_{all}$	Acc	$F1_{hem}$	$F1_{all}$
VGG16	80.01	78.05	81.05	75.25	72.10	78.91	70.09	65.52	74.21
VGG19	80.50	77.68	81.90	74.65	71.59	76.25	71.23	69.32	71.59
DenseNet121	81.23	79.52	82.54	77.13	77.32	80.58	73.39	70.62	75.43
DenseNet169	81.58	79.91	83.15	76.91	74.14	77.65	69.52	64.78	72.78
DenseNet201	80.90	78.02	83.09	78.39	73.92	80.32	71.63	68.59	73.80
AlexNet	**92.48**	90.91	94.15	88.91	87.14	91.50	80.25	78.79	82.71

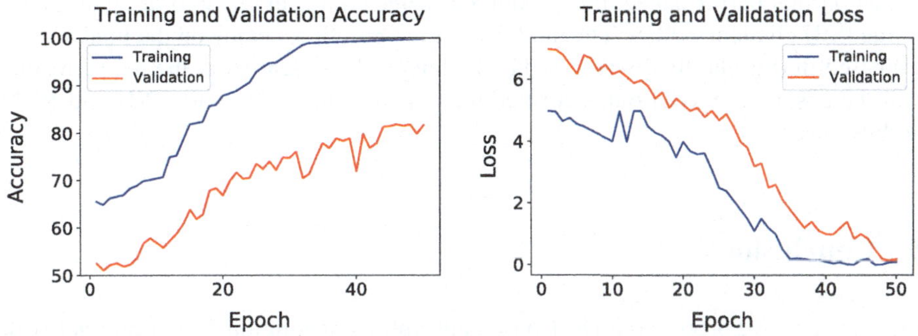

Fig. 4 Training and validation curves for **Phase 2** on test data

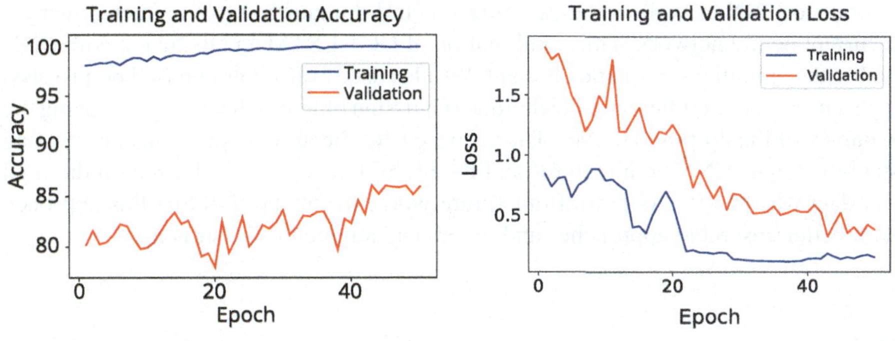

Fig. 5 Training and validation curves for **Phase 4** on test data

Finally, in **Phase 4**, we train the DCT-LSTM model. Once trained, this model is added to the AlexNet and LSTM-DENSE models trained in the preceding phases. The final classification decision is made by averaging the score of the three models in the ensemble.

This final model achieved 86.13% accuracy on test data from the second phase of the challenge.The training and validation curves for Phase 4 are plotted in Fig. 5. Table 2 shows the performance of the proposed models on validation and test data.

Table 2 Performance of different models on validation and test data from the second phase of the challenge

Model name	Acc	$F1_{hem}$	$F1_{all}$
Phase 2	81.95	80.30	82.91
Phase 3	83.81	80.29	85.25
Phase 4	**86.13**	83.12	87.58

Phase 2: LSTM-DENSE only. **Phase 3**: AlexNet + LSTM-DENSE. **Phase 4**: AlexNet + LSTM-DENSE + DCT-LSTM

The model in Phase 4 achieved the highest accuracy on test and validation data. Based on this performance, this model was selected as our entry to the final phase of the ISBI challenge 2019. The model achieved 86.6% accuracy on the final test set (released during the final week of the challenge). It is clear from the above results that the ensemble model outperformed the existing state-of-the-art CNN and RNN architectures.

5 Conclusions

In this paper, we proposed a DCT-based ensemble convolutional recurrent network architecture for the classification of normal versus malignant cells from ISBI 2019 challenge. The developed hybrid architecture utilizes the feature extracted using pretrained CNN as well as the dynamic spectral domain features extracted using a recurrent neural network. This combination of DCT-LSTM and its fusion with CNN makes the classifier robust and efficient. We also used crop contour based preprocessing step and data augmentation technique (Gaussian blur and shear) for increasing the accuracy of the proposed model. The proposed architecture outperforms the existing state-of-the-art CNN architectures and the highest accuracy it achieved on the final test data was 86.6%. As part of our future work, we intend to refine this approach with better ensemble approaches and novel data augmentation strategies.

References

1. Bi, L., Kim, J., Ahn, E., Kumar, A., Fulham, M., Feng, D.: Dermoscopic image segmentation via multistage fully convolutional networks. IEEE Trans. Biomed. Eng. **64**(9), 2065–2074 (2017)
2. Chougrad, H., Zouaki, H., Alheyane, O.: Deep convolutional neural networks for breast cancer screening. Comput. Methods Programs Biomed. **157**, 19–30 (2018)
3. Duggal, R., Gupta, A., Gupta, R.: Segmentation of overlapping/touching white blood cell nuclei using artificial neural networks. In: CME Series on Hemato-Oncopathology. AIIMS (2016)
4. Duggal, R., Gupta, A., Gupta, R., Mallick, P.: SD-layer: stain deconvolutional layer for CNNs in medical microscopic imaging. In: International Conference on Medical Image Computing and Computer-Assisted Intervention, pp. 435–443. Springer (2017)

5. Duggal, R., Gupta, A., Gupta, R., Wadhwa, M., Ahuja, C.: Overlapping cell nuclei segmentation in microscopic images using deep belief networks. In: Proceedings of the Tenth Indian Conference on Computer Vision, Graphics and Image Processing, p. 82. ACM (2016)
6. Gupta, A., Gupta, R., Kumar, L., Thakkar, N., Satpathy, D.: GCTI-SN: Geometry-Inspired Chemical and Tissue Invariant Stain Normalization of Microscopic Medical Images (2018)
7. Gupta, R., Mallick, P., Duggal, R., Gupta, A., Sharma, O.: Stain color normalization and segmentation of plasma cells in microscopic images as a prelude to development of computer assisted automated disease diagnostic tool in multiple myeloma. Clin. Lymphoma Myeloma Leukemia **17**(1), e99 (2017)
8. Hochreiter, S., urgen Schmidhuber, J., Elvezia, C.: Long short-term memory. Neural Comput. **9**(8), 1735–1780 (1997)
9. Huang, G., Liu, Z., Van Der Maaten, L., Weinberger, K.Q.: Densely connected convolutional networks. In: Proceedings of the IEEE Conference on Computer Vision and Pattern Recognition, pp. 4700–4708 (2017)
10. Kant, S., Kumar, P., Gupta, A., Gupta, R., et al.: LeukoNet: DCT-based CNN architecture for the classification of normal versus leukemic blasts in B-ALL cancer (2018). arXiv:1810.07961
11. Krizhevsky, A., Sutskever, I., Hinton, G.E.: ImageNet classification with deep convolutional neural networks. In: Advances in Neural Information Processing Systems, pp. 1097–1105 (2012)
12. Kumar, A., Kim, J., Lyndon, D., Fulham, M., Feng, D.: An ensemble of fine-tuned convolutional neural networks for medical image classification. IEEE J. Biomed. Health Inform. **21**(1), 31–40 (2017)
13. Li, Y., Zhu, R., Mi, L., Cao, Y., Yao, D.: Segmentation of white blood cell from acute lymphoblastic leukemia images using dual-threshold method. Comput. Math. Methods Med. **2016** (2016)
14. Nawaz, W., Ahmed, S., Tahir, A., Khan, H.A.: Classification of breast cancer histology images using ALEXNET. In: International Conference Image Analysis and Recognition, pp. 869–876. Springer (2018)
15. Negm, A.S., Hassan, O.A., Kandil, A.H.: A decision support system for acute Leukaemia classification based on digital microscopic images. Alexandria Eng. J. (2017)
16. Nguyen, L.D., Lin, D., Lin, Z., Cao, J.: Deep CNNs for microscopic image classification by exploiting transfer learning and feature concatenation. In: 2018 IEEE International Symposium on Circuits and Systems (ISCAS), pp. 1–5. IEEE (2018)
17. Simonyan, K., Zisserman, A.: Very deep convolutional networks for large-scale image recognition (2014). arXiv:1409.1556
18. Socher, R., Huval, B., Bath, B., Manning, C.D., Ng, A.Y.: Convolutional-recursive deep learning for 3D object classification. In: Advances in Neural Information Processing Systems, pp. 656–664 (2012)
19. Tajbakhsh, N., Shin, J.Y., Gurudu, S.R., Hurst, R.T., Kendall, C.B., Gotway, M.B., Liang, J.: Convolutional neural networks for medical image analysis: full training or fine tuning? IEEE Trans. Med. Imaging **35**(5), 1299–1312 (2016)
20. Wang, X., Jiang, W., Luo, Z.: Combination of convolutional and recurrent neural network for sentiment analysis of short texts. In: Proceedings of COLING 2016, the 26th International Conference on Computational Linguistics: Technical Papers, pp. 2428–2437 (2016)
21. Weir, E.G., Borowitz, M.J.: Flow cytometry in the diagnosis of acute leukemia. In: Seminars in Hematology, vol. 38, pp. 124–138. Elsevier (2001)
22. Zhang, L., Lu, L., Nogues, I., Summers, R.M., Liu, S., Yao, J.: DeepPap: deep convolutional networks for cervical cell classification. IEEE J. Biomed. Health Inform. **21**(6), 1633–1643 (2017)
23. Zuo, H., Fan, H., Blasch, E., Ling, H.: Combining convolutional and recurrent neural networks for human skin detection. IEEE Signal Process. Lett. **24**(3), 289–293 (2017)

Deep Learning for Classifying of White Blood Cancer

Yifan Ding, Yujia Yang and Yan Cui

Abstract Cell classification by computer assistant technique has become a popular topic recently. It is crucial to do early disease diagnosis with less cost. In order to find efficient, high accuracy computer assistant methods, The International Symposium on Biomedical Imaging (ISBI) held the classification of normal vs malignant cells (C-NMC) challenge 2019 for classifying B-ALL white blood cancer microscopic images. Our team deploys several state-of-the-art CNN architectures and uses an ensemble method named stacking to boost the final prediction performance, which helped to get the eighth place in the preliminary phase and tenth place in the final phase. Weighted F1 scores evaluated on our model were 0.8674 and 0.8552, for the preliminary and final phase, respectively. It is a relatively reasonable result in such an expertise required task.

Keywords Deep learning · Ensemble model · CNN

1 Introduction

Acute lymphoblastic leukemia (ALL) is a type of lymphoma cancers which is generated by the abnormal proliferation of white blood cells (WBCs) [1]. The word "acute" in ALL comes from the fact that the disease progresses rapidly and may

Y. Ding · Y. Yang · Y. Cui (✉)
Zhuhai 4DAGE Tech Co., Ltd., Zhuhai, China
e-mail: cuiyan@wyu.edu.cn

Y. Ding
e-mail: dingyifan@cgaii.com

Y. Yang
e-mail: yangyujia@cgaii.com

Y. Ding
Jinan University, Guangzhou, China

Y. Cui
Wuyi University, Jiangmen, China

A. Gupta and R. Gupta (eds.), *ISBI 2019 C-NMC Challenge: Classification in Cancer Cell Imaging*, Lecture Notes in Bioengineering,
https://doi.org/10.1007/978-981-15-0798-4_4

lead to death if no appropriate treatment is given. Therefore, standardized and accurate pathological diagnoses are essential to improve the overall survival rate for the patients diagnosed with ALL.

Nowadays, the visual examination of blood smears is one of the most basic and important methods for diagnosing ALL. In particular, the percentage of malignant cells is a major consideration for diagnosing ALL and is also helpful for early treatment [2]. However, the traditional method relies on manual observation and counting the number of malignant cells. With the increase in incidence rate of ALL, the limitations of the traditional method have been slowly revealed, including the lack of standardization and heavy reliance on the experience and judgment of the pathologists. To assist the pathologists, many centers make use of the flow cytometry to detect ALL. Although flow cytometry is available, it is very expensive, and people in rural areas normally have limited access to the equipment. Therefore, there has been growing interest in developing computer methods and programs to assist in the diagnosis of ALL.

The International Symposium on Biomedical Imaging (ISBI) held the classification of normal vs malignant cells (C-NMC) challenge 2019 to identify the top-performing computational analysis and support the system that can differentiate malignant B-lymphocytes from normal B-lymphocytes. Accordingly, we presented a deep learning-based approach to classify lymphocytes. Our approach empirically deployed several neural networks to generate the first stage prediction, later by an ensemble technique named stacking to boost the final prediction. Ultimately, we got the eighth place in the preliminary phase and tenth in the final phase by weighted F1 score.

2 Related Works

Recently, leveraging convolution neural network to perform imaging tasks has become popular, particularly in the biomedical field. Several works have proved that the prediction accuracy of deep learning methods is comparable to human expert. For example, Wang et al. [3] presented a deep learning-based method for identifying cancer metastases. They also proved that combining deep learning methods with the human pathologist's diagnosis can improve the accuracy of pathological diagnoses. Grewal et al. [4] described a deep learning approach called Recurrent Attention DenseNet (RADnet) for detecting brain hemorrhage from computed tomography scans. RADnet demonstrates 81.82% hemorrhage prediction accuracy at computed tomography level, which is near to radiologists. Esteva et al. [5] used an end-to-end neural network to classify skin lesions, demonstrating an artificial intelligence capable of classifying skin cancer with a level of competence comparable to dermatologists.

Moreover, the advancements in deep learning have enabled algorithms to surpass the performance of medical experts. Kamnitsas et al. [6] presented a three-dimensional (3D) convolutional neural network in brain lesion segmentation, and considered both local features and global contextual features. Their architecture improves over the currently published state-of-the-art on the 2013 BRATS benchmark. Voets et al. [7] applied deep learning to detect diabetic retinopathy and diabetic macular edema in retinal fundus photographs automatically. Rajpukar et al. [8] presented a 34-layer convolution neural network which exceeds the performance of board-certified cardiologists in detecting heart arrhythmias from electrocardiograms and exceeded the average cardiologist performance in both recall and precision.

Closest to our work is the previous work of Rahul et al. [9–11]. They proposed a method for segmentation of immature white blood cells from microscopic images. Besides, they proposed a stain deconvolutional layer to detect the blood cancer and obtain accuracy of 93.2% in the task of differentiating malignant immature white blood cells from normal white blood cells.

Inspired by the above works, we deploy several state-of-the-art network architectures on this task. Furthermore, we initialize the weights of all the networks from pretrained model on ImageNet [12], which is similar to the work of Rajpurkar et al. [13]. To further improve the accuracy of diagnosis of ALL, we boosted the prediction performance by leveraging different networks which was enlightened by Deng and Yu [14].

3 Approach

3.1 Data Preprocessing

Challenge dataset [9–11, 15, 16], also referred to as C-NMC dataset, has been segmented from the whole blood smear microscopic images, but they still contain some errors like standing noise and illumination. This problem has largely been fixed by stain normalization [15, 16].

Intuitively, considering that cell's position has no relationships with cell's class, we deploy random affine transformation at the first place. Rotation range of degrees from -180 to $+180$ translate shift factor randomly sampled from -0.05 to $+0.05$, and the scale factor is randomly sampled from 0.9 to 1.1, and all the images are flipped vertical–horizontal randomly with 50% chance. Then we center crop all images to 299 or 224, which depends on whether we deploy transfer learning on inception network or dense network. At last, we normalize all images with mean/std values at 0.5 or mean/std values calculated from ImageNet images, which also depends on network architecture.

3.2 Network Architecture

One of the most essential parts of deep learning is network architecture. We therefore select three different state-of-the-art network architectures to build our model after ablation experiments: InceptionV3, DenseNet121 and InceptionResNetV2. After training these three networks individually, we use an ensemble learning method named stacking to make a further and robust prediction.

InceptionV3 [17] uses multiple conv-kernel to get different receptive fields, and then concatenate those feature maps together in order to extract multi-scale features. Auxiliary loss is proposed for facilitating back propagation in such a deep architecture. The network architecture is shown in Fig. 1.

DenseNet [18] is a high efficient and memory saving architecture, which connects each layer to every other layer. For each layer, the feature maps of all preceding layers are concatenated together as inputs. The network architecture is illustrated in Fig. 2.

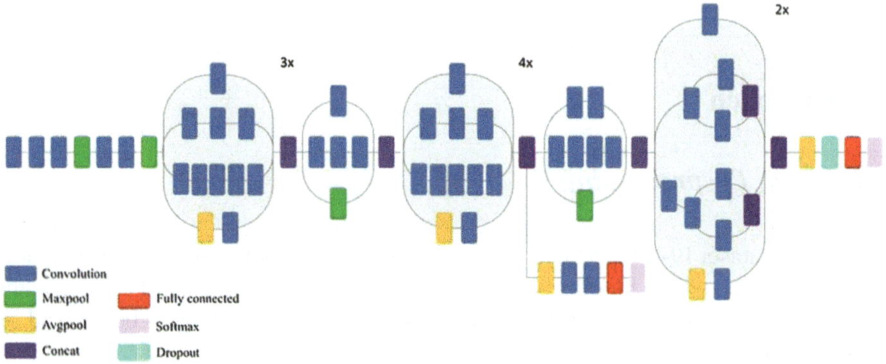

Fig. 1 The architecture of InceptionV3

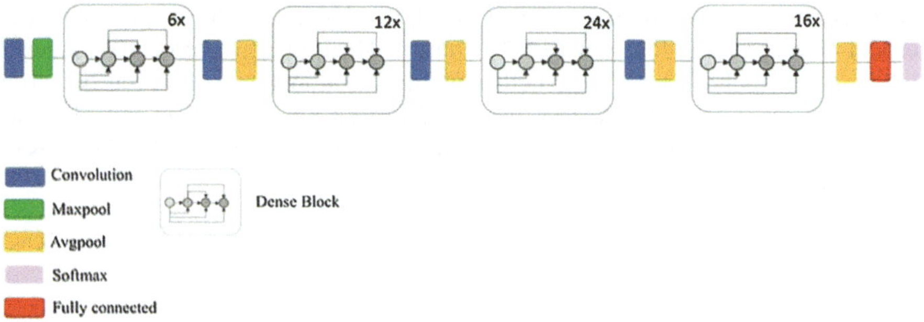

Fig. 2 The architecture of DenseNet121

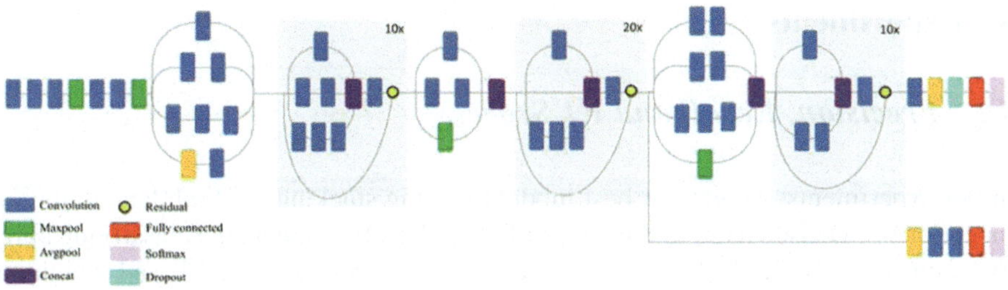

Fig. 3 The architecture of InceptionResnetV2

InceptionResNetV2 [19] is deeper than previous InceptionV3, with simplified inception blocks, fewer parallel towers and add repeated residual blocks. The network architecture is shown in Fig. 3.

3.3 Stacking

Stacking is an ensemble learning technique that combines multiple classification models via a meta-classifier [20]. We separate our training data into five parts, one part as validation set and rest for training, exactly like cross-validation. We get each five prediction logits of validation part from three different network architectures and merge them together as feature vectors. Then these feature vectors are trained by a selected meta-classifier for generating much stable prediction.

3.4 Training Details

We train all our networks on a single GTX 1080 GPU, using Adam optimizer with learning rate of 0.0001, and the loss function is cross-entropy:

$$L = -\sum_{x} p(x) \log q(x) \tag{1}$$

The biggest batch size allowed by our device is 48 (big batch size is benefit for BN). After training for base-level classifiers is finished, we ensemble all the three models together by adopting stacking with SVM-sigmoid kernel as our meta-classifier, which increases by 4% accuracy on our validation set. We use Pytorch, a popular open-source deep learning framework for all experiments. Note that all of our networks are pretrained on ImageNet and different architectures might have different hyper-parameters.

4 Experiments

4.1 Precision, Recall and F1 Score

In our experiments, we get our best model by using stacking method that combines InceptionV3, Densenet121 and InceptionResNetV2. To evaluate the classifying ability of our models, Table 1 gives weighted precision, weighted recall and weighted F1 score on each single model and stacking model.

4.2 AUC and ROC Curve

Area under the curve (AUC) and receiver operating characteristic (ROC) curve are important metrics for checking the performance of the classification model. We compare them on InceptionV3, Densenet121, InceptionResNetV2 and stacking model. In summary, the stacking technique, used to merge multi-models together, gives about 3% boost in AUC (Table 2). The ROC curve of stacking model is higher than any other single models in all ranges (see Fig. 4).

4.3 Subject- and Class-Level Accuracy

To evaluate the model stability and find further solution, we measure the subject- and class-level accuracy. In subject level, we find the accuracies of subject ID H36, H29, H35, H50, H34, H25 and H33 are less than 0.6, especially H25 is only 0.2. It

Table 1 Metrics on each single model and stacking model

Model	Precision	Weighted recall	Weight F1 score
Stacking	**0.8695**	**0.8653**	**0.8674**
Inceptionv3	0.8258	0.8265	0.8261
Densenet121	0.8399	0.8399	0.8347
InceptionResNetV2	0.7900	0.7937	0.7903

'bold' indicates the best performance in our ablation study

Table 2 AUC on each single model and stacking model

Model	AUC
Stacking	0.8315
Inceptionv3	0.8119
Densenet121	0.7804
InceptionResNetV2	0.7894

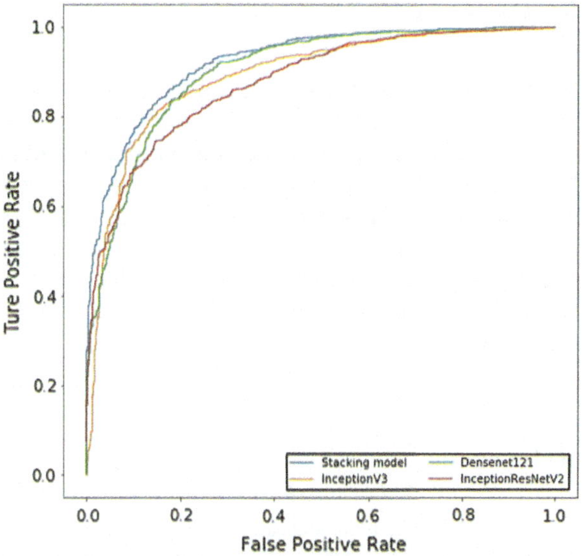

Fig. 4 The ROC curve of each model and stacking model

Table 3 Accuracy of cancer cells and normal cells

Class	Accuracy
Cancer	0.9325
Normal	0.7356

might be statistic bias because H25 has only 19 samples. Most of the low-accuracy subjects are cancer subjects, which are the same as the accuracy in the class level. The accuracy on cancer cells is 0.9325 and only 0.7356 on normal cells (Table 3). We have not found any good solution to increase the accuracy of normal cells. The accuracy of each subject is shown in Fig. 5.

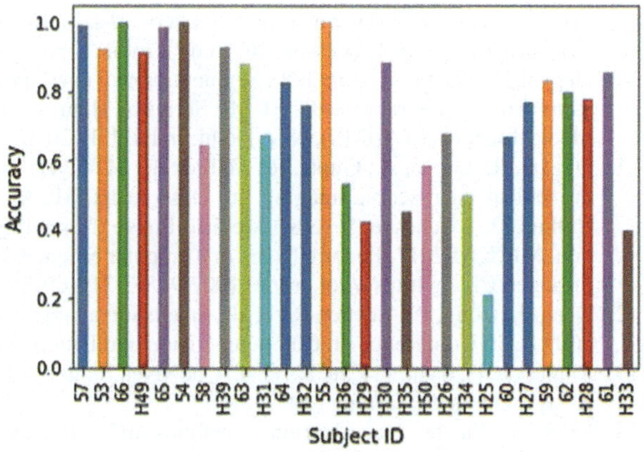

Fig. 5 The accuracy of each subject

5 Discussion

We have presented an ensemble neural network model for white blood cancer microscopic images classification. Our model gets weighted F1 score of 0.8552 and tenth place on the leaderboard. We demonstrate that stacking technique works well on deep learning models and performs better than any single model in our experiments. But we cannot solve the accuracy imbalance problem between cancer cells and normal cells. The accuracy on the normal cells is still very low. Our future work will try to find solutions for accuracy imbalance problem and explore other methods, such as Siamese network and metric learning, which were often used in one-shot task like face recognition.

References

1. Pui, C.H.: Acute lymphoblastic leukemia. Pediatr. Clin. North Am. **44**(4), 831 (1997)
2. Nazlibilek, S., Karacor, D., Ercan, T., et al.: Automatic segmentation, counting, size determination and classification of white blood cells. Measurement **55**, 58–65 (2014)
3. Wang, D., Khosla, A., Gargeya, R., et al.: Deep learning for identifying metastatic breast cancer (2016)
4. Grewal, M., Srivastava, M.M., Kumar, P., et al.: RADNET: radiologist level accuracy using deep learning for HEMORRHAGE detection in CT scans (2017)
5. Esteva, A., Kuprel, B., Novoa, R.A., et al.: Dermatologist-level classification of skin cancer with deep neural networks. Nature **542**(7639), 115–118 (2017)
6. Kamnitsas, K., Ledig, C., Newcombe, V.F.J., et al.: Efficient multi-scale 3D CNN with fully connected CRF for accurate brain lesion segmentation. Med. Image Anal. (2016). S1361841516301839
7. Voets, M., Møllersen, K., Bongo, L.A.: Replication study: development and validation of deep learning algorithm for detection of diabetic retinopathy in retinal fundus photographs (2018)
8. Rajpurkar, P., Hannun, A.Y., Haghpanahi, M., et al.: Cardiologist-level Arrhythmia detection with convolutional neural networks (2017)
9. Duggal, R., Gupta, A., Gupta, R., Wadhwa, M., Ahuja, C.: Overlapping cell nuclei segmentation in microscopic images using deep belief networks. In: Indian Conference on Computer Vision, Graphics and Image Processing (ICVGIP), India, December 2016
10. Duggal, R., Gupta, A., Gupta, R.: Segmentation of overlapping/touching white blood cell nuclei using artificial neural networks. CME Series on Hemato-Oncopathology, All India Institute of Medical Sciences (AIIMS), New Delhi, India, July 2016
11. Duggal, R., Gupta, A., Gupta, R., Mallick, P.: SD-layer: stain deconvolutional layer for CNNs in medical microscopic imaging. In: Descoteaux, M., Maier-Hein, L., Franz, A., Jannin, P., Collins, D., Duchesne, S. (eds.) Medical Image Computing and Computer-Assisted Intervention, MICCAI 2017. Lecture Notes in Computer Science, Part III, LNCS 10435, pp. 435–443. Springer, Cham. https://doi.org/10.1007/978-3-319-66179-7_50
12. Deng, J., Dong, W., Socher, R., et al.: ImageNet: a large-scale hierarchical image database. In: 2009 IEEE Conference on Computer Vision and Pattern Recognition. IEEE (2009)
13. Rajpurkar, P., Irvin, J., Zhu, K., et al.: CheXNet: radiologist-level pneumonia detection on chest X-rays with deep learning (2017)
14. Deng, L., Yu, D.: Deep learning: methods and applications. Found. Trends Signal Process. **7**(3), 197–387 (2014)

15. Gupta, A., Duggal, R., Gupta, R., Kumar, L., Thakkar, N., Satpathy, D.: GCTI-SN: Geometry-Inspired Chemical and Tissue Invariant Stain Normalization of Microscopic Medical Images. Under review
16. Gupta, R., Mallick, P., Duggal, R., Gupta, A., Sharma, O.: Stain color normalization and segmentation of plasma cells in microscopic images as a prelude to development of computer assisted automated disease diagnostic tool in multiple Myeloma. In: 16th International Myeloma Workshop (IMW), India, March 2017
17. Szegedy, C., Vanhoucke, V., Ioffe, S., Shlens, J., Wojna, Z.: Rethinking the inception architecture for computer vision. In: CVPR (2016)
18. Huang, G., Liu, Z., Weinberger, K.Q., Maaten, L.: Densely connected convolutional networks. In: CVPR (2017)
19. Szegedy, C., Ioffe, S., Vanhoucke, V.: Inception-v4, Inception-ResNet and the impact of residual connections on learning. In: CoRR (2016). arXiv:1602.07261
20. Breiman, L.: Stacked regressions. Mach. Learn. **24**(1), 49–64 (1996)

Ensemble Convolutional Neural Networks for Cell Classification in Microscopic Images

Tian Shi, Longshi Wu, Changhong Zhong, Ruixuan Wang and Weishi Zheng

Abstract In this challenge, we address the cell classification problem using deep convolutional neural networks (CNNs). For a better generalization of the CNN classifier, various data augmentation and preprocessing were tested and an ensemble of state-of-the-art CNNs was adopted. In addition, to check the stability of the CNN model, the Grad-CAM technique was used to visualize the most discriminative part of each cell when predicting the category of the cell image. Our model achieves an accuracy of 86.9% in the preliminary testing and 87.9% in the final testing.

Keywords Convolutional neural networks · Ensemble model · Cell classification

1 Introduction

Accurate classification of normal and malignant cells in microscopic images is challenging partially due to the high similarity between some of the malignant cells and normal ones. In this cell classification challenge, to improve the generalization of the final classifier, numerous experiments and preliminary evaluations were performed based on the released training and validation dataset. Consequently, we chose to

---

T. Shi, L. Wu and C. Zhong—are equally contributed.

T. Shi · L. Wu · C. Zhong · R. Wang (✉) · W. Zheng
School of Data and Computer Science, Sun Yat-sen University, Guangzhou, China
e-mail: wangruix5@mail.sysu.edu.cn

T. Shi
e-mail: shit6@mail2.sysu.edu.cn

L. Wu
e-mail: wulsh26@mail2.sysu.edu.cn

C. Zhong
e-mail: zhongchh7@mail2.sysu.edu.cn

W. Zheng
e-mail: wszheng@ieee.org

A. Gupta and R. Gupta (eds.), *ISBI 2019 C-NMC Challenge: Classification in Cancer Cell Imaging*, Lecture Notes in Bioengineering,
https://doi.org/10.1007/978-981-15-0798-4_5

ensemble multiple state-of-the-art CNNs as the final classifier. The details of the CNNs and the procedure of model training and testing will be introduced in Sect. 2 while the preliminary experimental evaluation will be reported in Sect. 4.

2 Method

2.1 *The Selected CNNs: SENet and PNASNet*

In the first phase of the challenge, multiple CNNs (including ResNet [1], VGG [2], and DenseNet [3]) were empirically evaluated and compared. After comprehensive experiments, we found that SENet and PNASNet performed best among all the CNN models, which actually confirmed the superior performance of the two models in the classification of natural images [4, 5].

In SENet, a "Squeeze-and-Excitation" (SE) block unit is added in parallel to one or more convolutional layers such that SENet can learn to adaptively focus on different feature channels at these CNN layers for different input images. In this challenge, we chose the SENet-154 model which was generated by adding the SE block to ResNet-154. Different from SENet, PNASNet is a novel CNN architecture automatically generated based on a sequential model-based optimization process. We applied the pretrained SENet and PNASNet models for this challenge task.

2.2 *Data Augmentation*

For the data preprocessing and augmentation part, pixel-wise normalization was first applied by subtracting the mean of all pixel's values over all training images and divided by the standard deviation of all pixel values. Then, as part of augmentation during model training, each image was randomly resized (rescaled with or without keeping aspect ratio) and rotated to generate more training data. In addition, a center crop was adopted to remove the surrounding background regions in each image. All the preprocessing and augmentations helped improve classification performance.

2.3 *Ensemble CNNs*

The Ensemble model is widely adopted in classification tasks because of its better generalization than single models. Here, we applied a 2-step ensemble process. First, for each test image and each CNN model, multiple augmented images were generated by applying random rotation to the image and each rotated image was predicted, thus resulting in multiple predictions for the same test image. The voting scheme was adopted from the multiple predictions for the prediction of the image by the CNN model. The same prediction procedure was performed for each CNN model. Then in the second step, the predictions from multiple CNNs were voted again for the final prediction of the test image by the ensemble model.

2.4 Grad-CAM for Visualizing

In this challenge task, to investigate how and why the CNN model works, Grad-CAM [6] was applied to visualize the attended regions in each test image during prediction by the model. With this investigation, we can check whether the model did focus on interesting cell regions during classification and find any potential incorrect attention (e.g., outside cell regions).

3 Related Work

Cell classification using deep convolutional networks. Convolutional auto-encoder neural network architecture [7] was proposed to intelligently learn the feature in an unsupervised way and classify it via a softmax classifier without a fully connected layer. A deep fully connected layer surpassed traditional machine learning methods (e.g., support vector machine and logistic regression) in a label-free cell classification problem when the features were extracted by optical loss and phase fusion [8]. Deep convolutional neural networks were compared with fisher linear discriminant and random forest, showing a better performance in single-cell classification problem [9]. Deep Pap [10] trained the convolutional network on nature images (e.g., ImageNet) and fine-tuned the model on the cervical cell dataset. Inception v3 [11] was applied on non-small cell classification and mutation prediction [12].

Modern deep convolutional architectures and ensemble methods. A deep residual network (ResNet) showed the effectiveness of deep convolutional networks. Batch normalization(BN) [13] improved gradient propagation by inserting normalization in each training batch. Inception methods [14] demonstrated the benefits of increasing the depth of the convolutional layer. Recent data modeling research has shown that ensemble methods have gained much popularity as they often perform better than individual models [15, 16].

4 Experiments

We perform three types of experiments on both the preliminary testing and final testing. The first and second experiment evaluated the effects of SENet and PNAS-Net separately (Sects. 4.1 and 4.2). The third experiment explores the impact of the number of votes on the final results (Sect. 4.3).

Table 1 Augmentation settings

Methods	Settings
Random resize	Scale ($0.80 \sim 1.2$), Ratio ($0.75 \sim 1.3333$)
Random crop	224×224
Random rotation	$(-180^\circ \sim 180^\circ)$
Normalize	True

In the preliminary testing phase, we trained our model with all initial training data which is obtained by combining three folders together. In the final testing phase, we put the validation set as a part of our training data but kept 20% of them for validation to avoid overfitting.

4.1 Evaluation of Preliminary Testing

The training dataset is composed of 10.6k 450×450 RGB images of two classes, with 7.2k images of malignant and 3.4k images of normal cells. There are about 1800 images for testing in this phase. In addition, we found that the obvious imbalance of the given data might be a problem while training. Hence, we set a class weight for two classes and they got a different weight in the process of calculating the loss. Many proportions of weights were adopted and compared. The adjustment of class weight might increase accuracy in a way but the recall and precision became unstable. Our group is still doing experiments to reveal the relationship between them so we used the default weight (1:1) for the following experiments.

On all training datasets, we follow the data augmentation described in Table 1. For each training sample, randomly resize first to generate a different scale of the image and crop a fixed-size area randomly. A cell image should be identified accurately no matter what direction should be captured. Consequently, we applied rotation in order to improve the robustness of the model.

In the part of testing, we not only did prediction by two models separately but also fused their results together and voted again. In this way, we believed that we made a duplicate confirmation on some controversial samples which were the key to the whole dataset. As shown in Fig. 1, the model fusing technique established a new maximum accuracy, improving the previous results by almost 1.5%. This suggests that our ensemble approach is suitable for this classification task. (Detailed experiments about ensemble voting and model fusing are shown in Sect. 4.3)

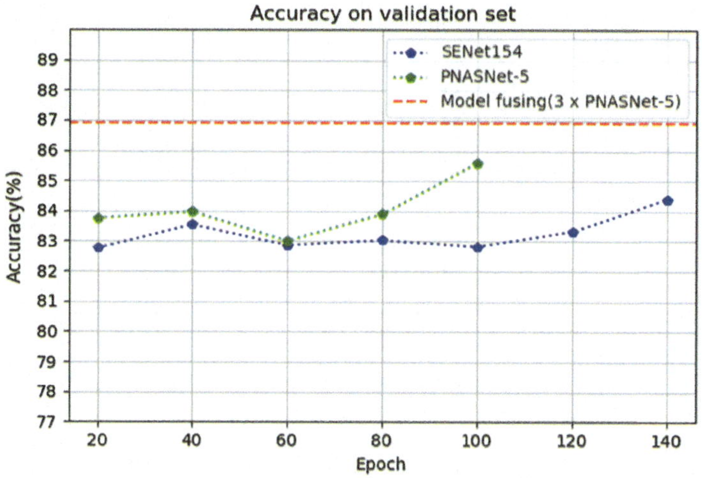

Fig. 1 The comparison between SENet154 and PNASNet-5 as well as the final result generated by model fusing (3 x PNASNet-5). SENet154 needs about 140 epochs to converge while PNASNet-5 needs 100

Table 2 Results in final testing

Methods	Score
3 x SENet154 + vote51	**87.98**

4.2 *Evaluation of Final Testing*

The final testing set consists of about 2500 samples with a size of 600 $\times$ 600. We trained the model as before but there was a little difference in testing. Due to the change of image size, we cropped the images at the center to generate images with a size of 450 $\times$ 450 before doing any data augmentation.

We could only submit our results twice which is the maximum limitation totally, so we did not get the results of two single models but only the results of ensemble voting and fusing. The results are shown in Table 2. Our approach reached the best score of 87.98 in the final testing.

4.3 *Comparison of Ensemble Voting*

We did more experiments on ensemble voting to explore the effect of the number of votes. Results are shown in Table 3. We used SENet154 as a basic model because it is much faster to train compared with PNASNet-5. The votes we set are 1, 11, 31 and 51. It is obvious that the more votes, the better the results.

Next, we tried more experiments to explore the effectiveness of combining both voting and fusing together. And restricted by the lack of computation resources, we

Table 3 Accuracy increases with the number of votes (SENet154)

Number of votes	Accuracy
1	84.4
11	85.0
31	85.3
51	**85.5**

Table 4 SENet154

Methods	Accuracy
SENet154	84.4
3 x SENet154	84.8
SENet154 + vote11	85.0
3 x SENet154 + vote11	**85.3**

Table 5 PNASNet-5

Methods	Accuracy
PNASNet-5	85.6
3 x PNASNet-5	86.9
PNASNet-5 + vote11	86.6
3 x PNASNet-5 + vote11	**87.9**

only did a few comparative tests but the results were enough to support our idea. We chose 11 as the number of votes, three trained models to fuse and used preliminary testing data as a validation set. Results are shown in Tables 4 and 5. Irrespective of using ensemble voting or model fusing, the results are all better than using the single model. In addition, there are additional slight improvements when using both of them at the same time.

5 Visualizing by Grad-CAM

Although the accuracy of classification between normal and malignant cells reaches a satisfying level, it may not be true that the model is intelligent enough to perceive the features in images as humans do. We are still curious about which part of the cell the CNNs are looking at. Is the model exactly understanding the images as professional doctors do? If true, we are glad to say that the model may get an opportunity to help in the process of diagnosing patients. However, if not true, the model will probably fail seriously in some unknown special cases.

In Fig. 2, the center part of the well-classified cell is focused on. However, if we force our model to classify it wrongly, the attention part becomes the edge of the cell. Obviously, that means our model has a good perception of these cells and is not exactly a "black box" anymore.

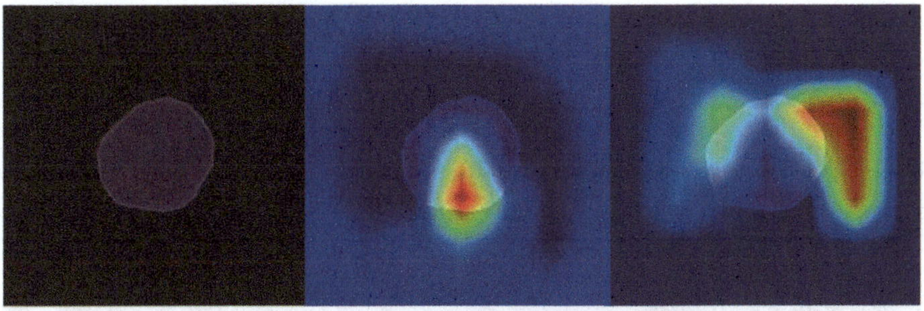

Fig. 2 For a well-classified cell (left), our model successfully focuses on the center part of the cell (middle). If we force the model to identify it wrongly, the attention part is moving away from the cell (right)

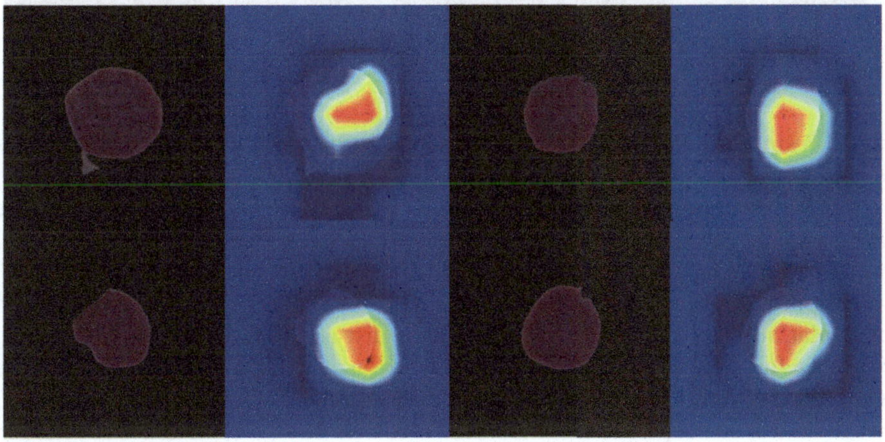

Fig. 3 Cells that are identified precisely

Other cases are also listed in Figs. 2 and 3. For those who are identified well, our model always focuses on the middle part of them. However, for those who are identified wrongly, our model shows failure in recognizing the kernel part. Hence, our model still can be optimized in some way (Fig. 4).

6 Conclusion

We introduced our strategy for the cell classification between normal and malignant cells that assemble our models' results together for voting and fusing. There are three key components of our model: (1) deep neural networks—SENet and PNASNet, (2) random resize and crop augmentation, and (3) ensemble voting combined with

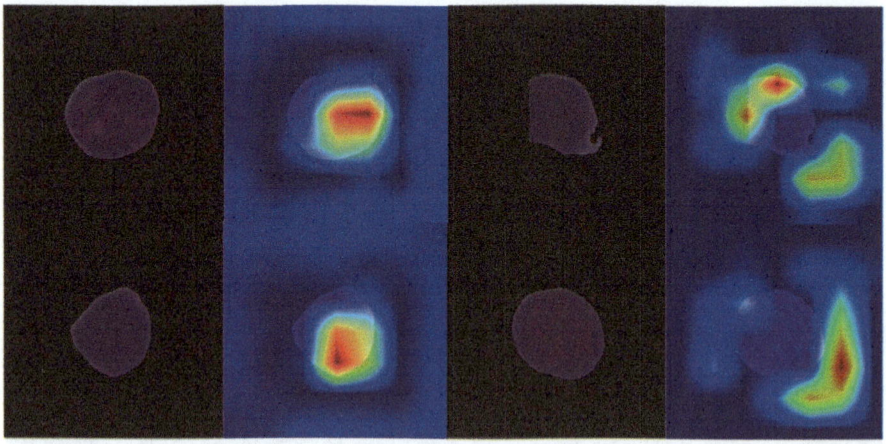

Fig. 4 Cells that are identified wrongly

model fusing. Results on preliminary testing and final testing show that our model is able to identify abnormal cells accurately and has good stability.

We also tried to explain how and why our CNNs work well using the technique of Grad-CAM. Most of the sensitive area of the cells is the center part of them. We, therefore, hypothesize that the model correctly puts the attention right on the cell.

Despite the promising results, cell classification problem is far from solved. In particular, an accuracy of 90% is not enough for disease diagnosis but only an assisted reference for doctors. In future work, we plan to analyze the effect of data imbalance and try to fully take advantage of the subject information, hoping that deep neural networks can be adopted in more an more scenarios of medical image analysis.

References

1. He, K., Zhang, X., Ren, S., Sun, J.: Deep residual learning for image recognition. In: Proceedings of the IEEE Conference on Computer Vision and Pattern Recognition, pp. 770–778 (2016)
2. Simonyan, K., Zisserman, A.: Very deep convolutional networks for large-scale image recognition. arXiv preprint arXiv:1409.1556 (2014)
3. Huang, G., Liu, Z., Van Der Maaten, L., Weinberger, K.Q.: Densely connected convolutional networks. In: Proceedings of the IEEE Conference on Computer Vision and Pattern Recognition, pp. 4700–4708 (2017)
4. Hu, J., Shen, L., Sun, G.: Squeeze-and-excitation networks. In: Proceedings of the IEEE Conference on Computer Vision and Pattern Recognition, pp. 7132–7141 (2018)
5. Liu, C., Zoph, B., Neumann, M., Shlens, J., Hua, W., Li, L.J., et al.: Progressive neural architecture search. In: Proceedings of the European Conference on Computer Vision (ECCV), pp. 19–34 (2018)

6. Selvaraju, R.R., Cogswell, M., Das, A., Vedantam, R., Parikh, D., Batra, D.: Grad-cam: visual explanations from deep networks via gradient-based localization. In: Proceedings of the IEEE International Conference on Computer Vision, pp. 618–626 (2017)
7. Cruz-Roa, A.A., Ovalle, J.E.A., Madabhushi, A., Osorio, F.A.G.: A deep learning architecture for image representation, visual interpretability and automated basal-cell carcinoma cancer detection. In: International Conference on Medical Image Computing and Computer-Assisted Intervention, pp. 403–410. Springer, Berlin (2013)
8. Chen, C.L., Mahjoubfar, A., Tai, L.C., Blaby, I.K., Huang, A., Niazi, K.R., Jalali, B.: Deep learning in label-free cell classification. Sci. Rep. **6**, 21471 (2016)
9. Drr, O., Sick, B.: Single-cell phenotype classification using deep convolutional neural networks. J. Biomol. Screen. **21**(9), 998–1003 (2016)
10. Zhang, L., Lu, L., Nogues, I., Summers, R.M., Liu, S., Yao, J.: DeepPap: deep convolutional networks for cervical cell classification. IEEE J. Biomed. Health Inform. **21**(6), 1633–1643 (2017)
11. Szegedy, C., Vanhoucke, V., Ioffe, S., Shlens, J., Wojna, Z.: Rethinking the inception architecture for computer vision. In: Proceedings of the IEEE Conference on Computer Vision and Pattern Recognition, pp. 2818–2826 (2016)
12. Coudray, N., Ocampo, P.S., Sakellaropoulos, T., Narula, N., Snuderl, M., Feny, D., Tsirigos, A.: Classification and mutation prediction from nonsmall cell lung cancer histopathology images using deep learning. Nat. Med. **24**(10), 1559 (2018)
13. Ioffe, S., Szegedy, C.: Batch normalization: Accelerating deep network training by reducing internal covariate shift. arXiv preprint arXiv:1502.03167 (2015)
14. Szegedy, C., Liu, W., Jia, Y., Sermanet, P., Reed, S., Anguelov, D., et al.: Going deeper with convolutions. In: Proceedings of the IEEE Conference on Computer Vision and Pattern Recognition, pp. 1–9 (2015)
15. Yang, P., Hwa Yang, Y., Zhou, B.B., Zomaya, A.Y.: A review of ensemble methods in bioinformatics. Curr. Bioinform. **5**(4), 296–308 (2010)
16. Opitz, D., Maclin, R.: Popular ensemble methods: an empirical study. J. Artif. Intell. Res. **11**, 169–198 (1999)
17. Gupta, A., Duggal, R., Gupta, R., Kumar, L., Thakkar, N., Satpathy, D.: GCTI-SN: geometry-inspired chemical and tissue invariant stain normalization of microscopic medical images (under review)
18. Gupta, R., Mallick, P., Duggal, R., Gupta, A., Sharma, O.: Stain color normalization and segmentation of plasma cells in microscopic images as a prelude to development of computer assisted automated disease diagnostic tool in multiple Myeloma. In: 16th International Myeloma Workshop (IMW), India (2017)
19. Duggal, R., Gupta, A., Gupta, R., Wadhwa, M., Ahuja, C.: Overlapping cell nuclei segmentation in microscopic images using deep belief networks. In: Indian Conference on Computer Vision, Graphics and Image Processing (ICVGIP), India (2016)
20. Duggal, R., Gupta, A., Gupta, R.: Segmentation of overlapping/touching white blood cell nuclei using artificial neural networks. CME Series on Hemato-Oncopathology, All India Institute of Medical Sciences (AIIMS), New Delhi, India (2016)
21. Duggal, R., Gupta, A., Gupta, R., Mallick, P.: SD-Layer: stain deconvolutional layer for CNNs in medical microscopic imaging. In: Descoteaux, M., Maier-Hein, L., Franz, A., Jannin, P., Collins, D., Duchesne, S. (eds.) Medical Image Computing and Computer-Assisted Intervention MICCAI 2017, MICCAI 2017. Lecture Notes in Computer Science, Part III, LNCS 10435, pp. 435–443. Springer, Cham (2017). https://doi.org/10.1007/978-3-319-66179-7_50

Acute Lymphoblastic Leukemia Classification from Microscopic Images Using Convolutional Neural Networks

Jonas Prellberg and Oliver Kramer

Abstract Examining blood microscopic images for leukemia is necessary when expensive equipment for flow cytometry is unavailable. Automated systems can ease the burden on medical experts for performing this examination and may be especially helpful to quickly screen a large number of patients. We present a simple, yet effective classification approach using a ResNeXt convolutional neural network with Squeeze-and-Excitation modules. The approach was evaluated in the C-NMC online challenge and achieves a weighted $F1$-score of 88.91 % on the test set. Code is available at https://github.com/jprellberg/isbi2019cancer.

1 Introduction

Acute lymphoblastic leukemia (ALL) is a blood cancer that is characterized by the proliferation of abnormal lymphoblast cells, eventually leading to the accumulation of a lethal number of leukemia cells [12]. If ALL is diagnosed in an early stage, treatment is possible. Diagnosis is typically performed using a complete blood count and morphological analysis of cells under a microscope by a medical expert. Flow cytometry can replace this manual work but requires expensive equipment which is not available everywhere. Therefore, automated systems that can perform diagnosis using comparatively low-cost microscopic images provide a great advantage.

To further research in this direction, public datasets are necessary to compare different approaches and track the state-of-the-art. A popular example for single-cell ALL classification is ALL-IDB2 [9] but with only 260 images of white blood cells, the dataset is too small to properly take advantage of recent deep learning approaches. In 2018, a new dataset with more than 10,000 training images and a separate test set of normal B-lymphoid precursors and malignant B-lymphoblasts has been released

J. Prellberg (✉) · O. Kramer
University of Oldenburg, Oldenburg, Germany
e-mail: jonas.prellberg@uni-oldenburg.de

O. Kramer
e-mail: oliver.kramer@uni-oldenburg.de

A. Gupta and R. Gupta (eds.), *ISBI 2019 C-NMC Challenge: Classification in Cancer Cell Imaging*, Lecture Notes in Bioengineering,
https://doi.org/10.1007/978-981-15-0798-4_6

as an online challenge[1] open to the public. The large size of this new dataset allows creating improved classifiers based on deep neural networks and also provides a more reliable comparison of competing approaches.

In this work, we present our approach to the classification of healthy and malignant cells on the mentioned dataset using a convolutional neural network. In Sect. 2, the dataset is described in more detail and our data augmentation strategy is outlined. The convolutional neural network, a ResNeXt variant with Squeeze-and-Excitation modules, is presented in Sect. 3. In Sect. 4 we describe the training process and show experimental results. A summary of the related work and a conclusion follow.

2 Dataset

The challenge dataset [2–6], hereafter referred to as C-NMC dataset, contains images of white blood cells taken from 154 individual subjects, 84 of which exhibit ALL. Table 1 provides a detailed breakdown of the number of subjects and cells in the training and test sets. The dataset is imbalanced with about twice as many ALL cells as normal cells.

Each image has a resolution of 450×450 pixels and contains only a single cell as a consequence of preprocessing steps applied by the dataset authors: An automated segmentation algorithm has been used to separate the cells from the background. Each pixel that was determined not to be part of the cell is colored completely black. However, since the segmentation algorithm is not perfect, there are instances where parts of the cell are inadvertently colored black or a superfluous background is included. Additionally, all images have been preprocessed with a stain-normalization procedure that performs white-balancing and fixes errors introduced due to variations in the staining chemical [6]. See Fig. 1 for example images from the dataset.

Even though the dataset contains more than 10,000 images, several data augmentation techniques can be applied to increase the amount of training data further and improve the training of our convolutional neural network. Since microscopic images are invariant to flips and rotations, we perform horizontal and vertical flips with 50 % probability each and rotations with an angle from [0, 360) degrees chosen uniformly at random. Since convolutional neural networks with pooling operations or strides larger than one are not perfectly translation invariant, we also perform random translations of up to 20 % of each side length in horizontal and vertical directions.

We do not randomly scale the images because cell size may be a diagnostic factor to differentiate between ALL and normal cells [1]. Furthermore, we do not apply any brightness or color augmentation due to this dataset's stain-normalization preprocessing. Both data augmentation methods are commonly used but would lead to an unnecessary distribution shift between the training and test set on this specific dataset.

---

[1] https://competitions.codalab.org/competitions/20395.

Table 1 Composition of the dataset. The test set is unreleased and can only be evaluated against using an online service so its composition is unknown

Dataset part	ALL subjects	Normal subjects	ALL cells	Normal cells
Train	47	26	7272	3389
Preliminary test	13	15	1219	648
Final test	9	8	?	?

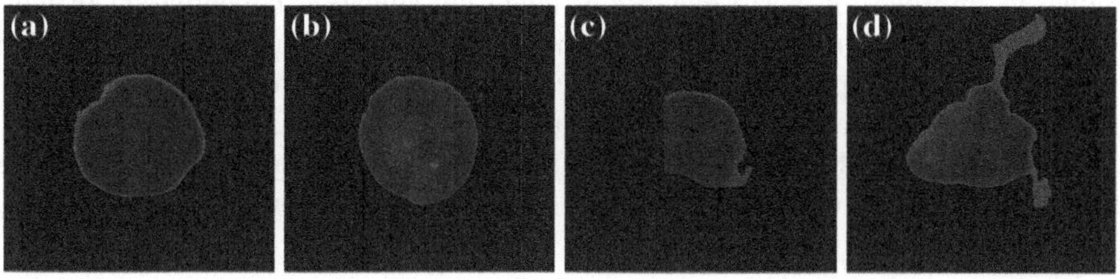

Fig. 1 Example images taken from the training set. **a** ALL cell. **b** Normal cell. **c** ALL cell with part of the cell cut off due to an imperfect segmentation. **d** Normal cell with superfluous background due to an imperfect segmentation

Additionally, the images are center-cropped to 300 × 300 pixels to decrease the dimensionality of the input data. This will generally make learning a classifier faster and easier. Even though the cropping discards large parts of the image, it has no effect on the classification accuracy because only very few cells are actually larger than this crop. In many cases, images that are not completely black outside of the crop are segmentation failures that include parts of the background.

3 Network Architecture

Image classification benchmarks have driven the creation of many powerful convolutional neural network architectures. We pick one of the recent top-performing networks, an ResNeXt50 [18], as our base model. The network consists of five convolutional stages with spatial downsampling by a factor of 2 in-between stages, followed by global average pooling and a linear classifier. Each stage is made from stacked building blocks, each of which computes a function of the form

$$x' = x + \sum_{i=1}^{C} \mathcal{T}_i(x)$$

where C is called the cardinality that controls the number of parallel paths in a block and $\mathcal{T}_i(x)$ is a function that projects x into a lower dimensional space, transforms it and projects back into a space of the original dimensionality. The functions $\mathcal{T}_i(x)$

are implemented using a sequence of 1×1, 3×3 and 1×1 convolutional layers. The block function is modified to

$$x' = x + \mathsf{SE}\left(\sum_{i=1}^{C} \mathcal{T}_i(x)\right)$$

where SE is the Squeeze-and-Excitation operation introduced in [7], which has been shown to improve the performance on image classification benchmarks. In general, the SE operation learns a channel-wise rescaling of feature maps. First, global average pooling is applied to the input feature map in order to spatially aggregate the information of each channel. The resulting vector is fed into a two-layer fully connected network that outputs scale factors. These factors are then used to scale each channel of the original input feature map. More details on the SE-ResNeXt50 architecture can be found in [7].

4 Experiments

The previously described network architecture is used to classify the C-NMC dataset. Since the dataset is imbalanced, the overall accuracy can be misleading and we report accuracy, sensitivity and specificity as well as weighted $F1$-scores, weighted precision, and weighted recall. For sensitivity and specificity, the ALL class is regarded as the positive class. Furthermore, because the data is from multiple subjects, we report subject-level accuracies.

Hyperparameters for the training procedure have been chosen by validating on the preliminary test set. The chosen hyperparameters are used for multiple training runs with different random seeds and the best model according to the $F1$-score on the preliminary test set is selected for our competition entry. Final results on the test set are taken from the online challenge leaderboard.

4.1 Training and Testing

The network is pretrained on ImageNet [15] and then fine-tuned on the C-NMC training set. The loss function is the weighted binary cross-entropy

$$l(y, \hat{y}) = wy \ln(\sigma(\hat{y})) + (1 - y) \ln(1 - \sigma(\hat{y}))$$

where σ is the sigmoid function, y is the true label, $\hat{y}$ is the network output, and $w = n_{\mathrm{n}}/n_{\mathrm{p}}$ is the ratio of negative to positive examples in the training set. The weight w helps to deal with the class imbalance present in the dataset.

Table 2 Results on the preliminary test set over 24 training runs using the best model of each run measured by $F1$-score

	Min.	Mean ± Std.	Max.		Min.	Mean ± Std.	Max.
Accuracy	86.40	87.96 ± 0.90	89.88	$F1$-score	86.28	87.89 ± 0.90	89.81
Sensitivity	88.43	92.01 ± 1.44	94.50	Precision	86.27	87.91 ± 0.90	89.81
Specificity	75.31	80.36 ± 2.39	84.72	Recall	86.40	87.96 ± 0.90	89.88

The network is fine-tuned for six epochs using Adam [8] with a batch size of 16. The learning rate is decayed using a step function that starts at $\eta_{\text{base}} = 1$ and is divided by 10 every two epochs. This learning rate is multiplied with factors specific to the part of the network that it is applied to the following: The first and second stages[2] have an effective learning rate of $\eta_{12} = 10^{-6}\eta_{\text{base}}$, the third to fifth stages use $\eta_{345} = 10^{-4}\eta_{\text{base}}$, and the last fully connected layer uses $\eta_{\text{fc}} = 10^{-2}\eta_{\text{base}}$.

This results in lower effective learning rates in the earlier layers of the network and is desirable because the network is initialized with weights from ImageNet pretraining. These have been shown to contain generally useful image filters in the lowest layers [19], and continuing to optimize these weights on a small dataset with large learning rates will degrade these general filters.

During inference, we present eight rotated versions of each image and average the network output to further improve classification results.

4.2 Model Selection

We find that results are sensitive to the random seed, despite all networks starting from the same weight initialization due to the pretraining. Therefore, we conduct 24 training runs with different random seeds and measure the $F1$-score on the preliminary test set over the course of the training. We collect the 24 model checkpoints that have the highest $F1$-scores in their respective training run and report results in Table 2.

The best model achieves an $F1$-score of 89.81 % on the preliminary test set. Figure 2 shows the evolution of loss and $F1$-score during its training process while Fig. 3 shows cell classification accuracy grouped by subject. Overall, the classification for healthy subjects is worse because the specificity is comparatively low. Consequently, false-positives can be expected when using the network for the diagnosis of patients. Still, false-positives are preferable to false-negatives when trying to diagnose cancer with an automated method.

[2] Stage refers to a stack of building blocks that operate on the same spatial resolution as described in Sect. 3 and [18].

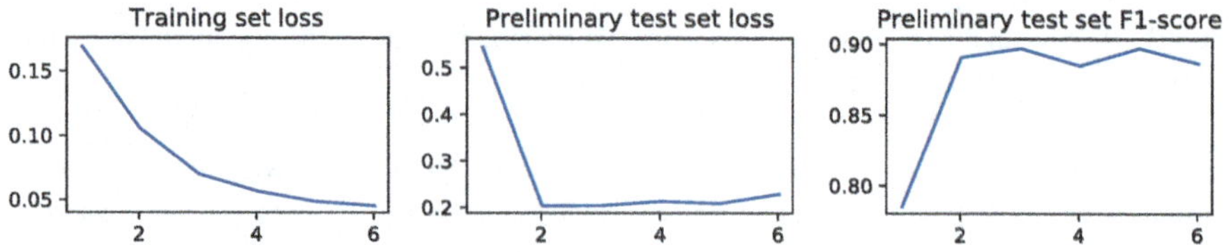

Fig. 2 Training and validation curves of the best model after each training epoch. The model achieves the maximum $F1$-score after the fifth training epoch

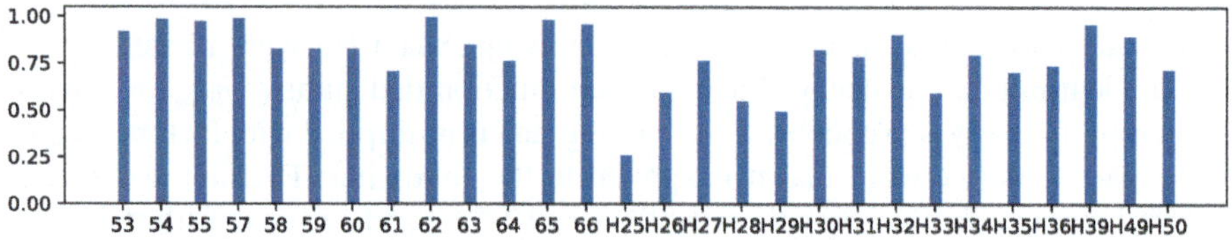

Fig. 3 Subject-level cell classification accuracy on the preliminary test set using the best model. Subjects with the prefix H are healthy

4.3 Results on the Final Test Set

We use the selected model to classify the final test set and submit the result to the online evaluation service. The model achieves a weighted $F1$-score of 88.91 %.

4.4 Ablation Studies

The main design choices we made for the training and testing procedures are layer-specific learning rates and test-time rotations. In order to show their impact, we perform two ablation studies:

NOROT The training procedure is unchanged but during testing, the images are only presented in their original orientation.

NOSPECLR During training, every layer has an effective learning rate of $\eta_{\text{all}}\eta_{\text{base}}$ while still using the scheduled decay for η_{base} as described previously. We test $\eta_{\text{all}} \in \{10^{-3}, 10^{-4}, 10^{-5}\}$ and report results for the best setting $\eta_{\text{all}} = 10^{-4}$. The testing procedure is unchanged.

Figure 4 shows results on the preliminary test set for our proposed setting (PROPOSAL) and the two ablation studies. As expected, both ablations decrease performance in terms of all considered metrics. Not using test-time rotations significantly ($p < 0.001$, one-sided Mann–Whitney U test) decreases the mean $F1$-score from 87.89 ± 0.90 % to 86.92 ± 0.81 %. The influence of layer-wise learning rates is significant ($p < 0.002$) but smaller: A constant learning rate for all layers decreases the mean $F1$-score to 87.20 ± 0.70 %.

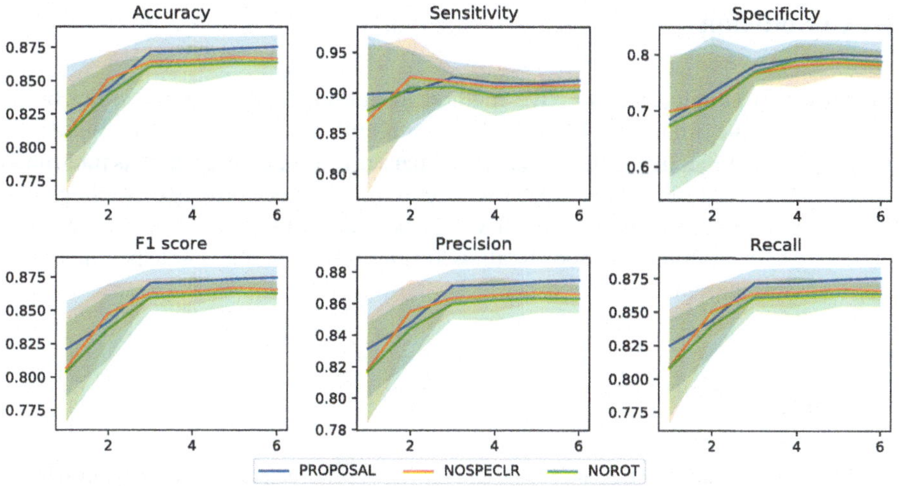

Fig. 4 Metrics on the preliminary test set measured after each training epoch for the proposed setting and the two ablation studies. Lines display the mean over 24 training runs and the shaded area marks one standard deviation. Best viewed electronically and zoomed in

5 Related Work

Previous work on automated ALL diagnosis from images can roughly be divided into more recent approaches that use convolutional neural networks as feature extractors and older approaches that use handcrafted features.

CNN features. Rehman et al. [14] classify ALL subtypes on a private dataset of 330 images using a pretrained AlexNet and fine-tuning. Shafique and Tehsin [16] classify ALL subtypes on ALL-IDB augmented with 50 private images, also using a pretrained AlexNet and fine-tuning. Vogado et al. [17] classify ALL on ALL-IDB using a number of different pretrained CNNs as fixed feature extractors. From these CNN features, the most informative ones are selected using PCA and finally, the classification is performed with an ensemble of SVM, MLP, and random forest.

Handcrafted features. Putzu and Ruberto [13] use ALL-IDB and classify a number of handcrafted features like area, compactness, roundness or area ratio between the cytoplasm and nucleus with an SVM. Mohapatra et al. [11] and Madhloom et al. [10] both use (different) private datasets and classify using an ensemble of naive Bayes, KNN, MLP, SVM, and a KNN classifier, respectively.

All works report good results but it is hardly possible to compare them because the private datasets are unavailable and even on the public ALL-IDB dataset, researchers employ their own evaluation procedures. Furthermore, in all cases the employed datasets are small, containing a couple of hundred images at most. It is important to have a large dataset that can be used to track the state-of-the-art and we hope that this role can be filled by the C-NMC dataset.

6 Conclusion

We present a simple, yet effective method to automatically classify white blood cell microscopic images into normal B-lymphoid precursors and malignant B-lymphoblasts. A recent convolutional neural network architecture which is fine-tuned on the C-NMC dataset achieves promising classification performance. We hope that the dataset authors release a version with raw images that have not been preprocessed by their in-house methods to allow further research that is not specific to this preprocessing pipeline.

References

1. Chiaretti, S., Zini, G., Bassan, R.: Diagnosis and subclassification of acute lymphoblastic leukemia. Mediterranean J. Hematol. Infect. Dis. **6**(1), e2014073–e2014073 (2014). https://www.ncbi.nlm.nih.gov/pubmed/25408859
2. Duggal, R., Gupta, A., Gupta, R.: Segmentation of overlapping/touching white blood cell nuclei using artificial neural networks. In: CME Series on Hemato-Oncopathology. All India Institute of Medical Sciences (AIIMS), New Delhi, India (2016)
3. Duggal, R., Gupta, A., Gupta, R., Mallick, P.: Sd-layer: stain deconvolutional layer for CNNS in medical microscopic imaging. In: Descoteaux, M., Maier-Hein, L., Franz, A., Jannin, P., Collins, D.L., Duchesne, S. (eds.) Medical Image Computing and Computer Assisted Intervention (MICCAI 2017), pp. 435–443. Springer International Publishing, Cham (2017)
4. Duggal, R., Gupta, A., Gupta, R., Wadhwa, M., Ahuja, C.: Overlapping cell nuclei segmentation in microscopic images using deep belief networks. In: Proceedings of the Tenth Indian Conference on Computer Vision, Graphics and Image Processing, pp. 82:1–82:8. ICVGIP '16, ACM, New York, NY, USA (2016). https://doi.org/10.1145/3009977.3010043
5. Gupta, A., Duggal, R., Gupta, R., Kumar, L., Thakkar, N., Satpathy, D.: GCTI-SN: geometry-inspired chemical and tissue invariant stain normalization of microscopic medical images (Under review)
6. Gupta, R., Mallick, P., Duggal, R., Gupta, A., Sharma, O.: Stain color normalization and segmentation of plasma cells in microscopic images as a prelude to development of computer assisted automated disease diagnostic tool in multiple myeloma. Clin. Lymphoma Myeloma Leuk. **17**(1), e99 (18 Mar 2019) (2017)
7. Hu, J., Shen, L., Sun, G.: Squeeze-and-excitation networks. In: The IEEE Conference on Computer Vision and Pattern Recognition (CVPR) (2018)
8. Kingma, D.P., Ba, J.: Adam: a method for stochastic optimization. In: The International Conference on Learning Representations (ICLR '15) (2015)
9. Labati, R.D., Piuri, V., Scotti, F.: All-IDB: the acute lymphoblastic leukemia image database for image processing. In: 2011 18th IEEE International Conference on Image Processing, pp. 2045–2048 (2011). https://doi.org/10.1109/ICIP.2011.6115881
10. Madhloom, H.T., Kareem, S.A., Ariffin, H.: A robust feature extraction and selection method for the recognition of lymphocytes versus acute lymphoblastic leukemia. In: 2012 International Conference on Advanced Computer Science Applications and Technologies (ACSAT), pp. 330–335 (2012). https://doi.org/10.1109/ACSAT.2012.62
11. Mohapatra, S., Patra, D., Satpathy, S.: An ensemble classifier system for early diagnosis of acute lymphoblastic leukemia in blood microscopic images. Neural Comput. Appl. **24**(7), 1887–1904 (2014). https://doi.org/10.1007/s00521-013-1438-3
12. Pui, C.H.: Acute Lymphoblastic Leukemia, pp. 39–43. Springer, Berlin (2017). https://doi.org/10.1007/978-3-662-46875-3_57

13. Putzu, L., Ruberto, C.D.: White blood cells identification and classification from leukemic blood image. In: International Work-Conference on Bioinformatics and Biomedical Engineering, IWBBIO 2013, Granada, Spain, 18–20 Mar 2013. Proceedings, pp. 99–106 (2013)
14. Rehman, A., Abbas, N., Saba, T., Rahman, S.I.U., Mehmood, Z., Kolivand, H.: Classification of acute lymphoblastic leukemia using deep learning. Microsc. Res. Tech. **81**(11), 1310–1317 (2018). https://doi.org/10.1002/jemt.23139
15. Russakovsky, O., Deng, J., Su, H., Krause, J., Satheesh, S., Ma, S., Huang, Z., Karpathy, A., Khosla, A., Bernstein, M., Berg, A.C., Fei-Fei, L.: ImageNet large scale visual recognition challenge. Int. J. Comput. Vis. (IJCV) **115**(3), 211–252 (2015). https://doi.org/10.1007/s11263-015-0816-y
16. Shafique, S., Tehsin, S.: Acute lymphoblastic leukemia detection and classification of its subtypes using pretrained deep convolutional neural networks. Technol. Cancer Res. Treat. **17**, 1533033818802789 (2018). https://doi.org/10.1177/1533033818802789 (pMID: 30261827)
17. Vogado, L.H.S., Veras, R.D.M.S., Andrade, A.R., Araujo, F.H.D.D., e. Silva, R.R.V., Aires, K.R.T.: Diagnosing leukemia in blood smear images using an ensemble of classifiers and pretrained convolutional neural networks. In: 2017 30th SIBGRAPI Conference on Graphics, Patterns and Images (SIBGRAPI), pp. 367–373 (2017). https://doi.org/10.1109/SIBGRAPI.2017.55
18. Xie, S., Girshick, R., Dollar, P., Tu, Z., He, K.: Aggregated residual transformations for deep neural networks. In: The IEEE Conference on Computer Vision and Pattern Recognition (CVPR) (2017)
19. Yosinski, J., Clune, J., Bengio, Y., Lipson, H.: How transferable are features in deep neural networks? In: Proceedings of the 27th International Conference on Neural Information Processing Systems, Vol. 2, pp. 3320–3328 (2014). NIPS'14, MIT Press, Cambridge, MA, USA, http://dl.acm.org/citation.cfm?id=2969033.2969197

Toward Automated Classification of B-Acute Lymphoblastic Leukemia

Rahul Kulhalli, Chinmay Savadikar and Bhushan Garware

Abstract We present an automated approach of classifying a stain-normalized white blood cell as being either a malignant (B-ALL) cell or a healthy (HEM) cell. We apply various data augmentations to the images in order to compensate for the class imbalance. As our primary approach, we use the ResNeXt101 Convolutional Neural Network architecture and "cut" it at various points in the network. We show that an ensemble of the same ResNeXt101 model trained for varying durations and a change in the decision threshold boundary lead to better performance as compared to individual model performances. Our final ensemble model leads to a weighted F1 score of 0.825 on the online preliminary test set. After training on the entire training data and validating in the preliminary test set, ResNeXt50 and ResNeXt101 achieve weighted F1 scores of 0.857 and 0.849 on the preliminary test set, respectively.

Keywords ISBI 2019 · Medical imaging · Convolutional neural networks · Classification · Ensembles

---

Supported by Persistent Systems Ltd.
Chinmay Savadikar, Rahul Kulhalli—Equal Contribution.

R. Kulhalli (✉) · C. Savadikar · B. Garware
Persistent Systems Ltd, Pune, India
e-mail: rahul_kulhalli@persistent.com
URL: https://www.persistent.com

C. Savadikar
e-mail: chinmay_savadikar@persistent.com

B. Garware
e-mail: bhushan_garware@persistent.com

A. Gupta and R. Gupta (eds.), *ISBI 2019 C-NMC Challenge: Classification in Cancer Cell Imaging*, Lecture Notes in Bioengineering,
https://doi.org/10.1007/978-981-15-0798-4_7

1 Introduction

Convolutional Neural Networks (CNNs) are proven to be extremely useful for a variety of imaging tasks such as object recognition, object detection, and segmentation [1–3]. This is attributed to the ability of CNNs to learn parameters to extract features that are most suitable for the task at hand. Since the application of CNNs for the ImageNet challenge in 2012 [4], there has been a steady performance gain due to development in CNN architectures [5–11], aided in part by the introduction of Batch Normalization [12].

However, CNNs require a large amount of data to generalize well, typically in the order of a million samples, making their application to small datasets difficult. This limitation can be addressed using transfer learning, where a network is first trained on a different, larger dataset and the parameters are reused/tuned for the target dataset.

We approached this classification task in two ways by considering the data as identical and independently distributed (i.i.d) and considering the images of the same patient to be dependent on some factor (i.e., not independent of each other). In both cases, we used transfer learning with fine-tuning.

1.1 Dataset

This dataset was acquired from the ISBI 2019 [13–17], a competition for Classification of Normal versus Malignant Cells in B-ALL White Blood Cancer Microscopic Images, organized by CodaLab. The dataset for Phase 1 consisted of data provided in three folds—fold 0, fold 1, and fold 2—all containing two classes—ALL (Acute Lymphoblastic Leukemia) and HEM (Healthy). The class distributions were approximately consistent across the three folds. This brings into picture the first challenge—class imbalance. Figures 1a–c show the class distributions for the three folds.

Each fold has a set of patients (denoted by IDs), and each patient has a set of associated cell images. The second challenging aspect of the data is seen here—each fold has a varying number of patients, and each patient has a varying set of images.

2 Non-i.i.d. Assumption

2.1 Data Splitting

We combined all the folds and used 70% of the total patients for training, 15% for validation, and 15% for testing. While splitting the data, we maintained the class distribution in each set. No data augmentation was used.

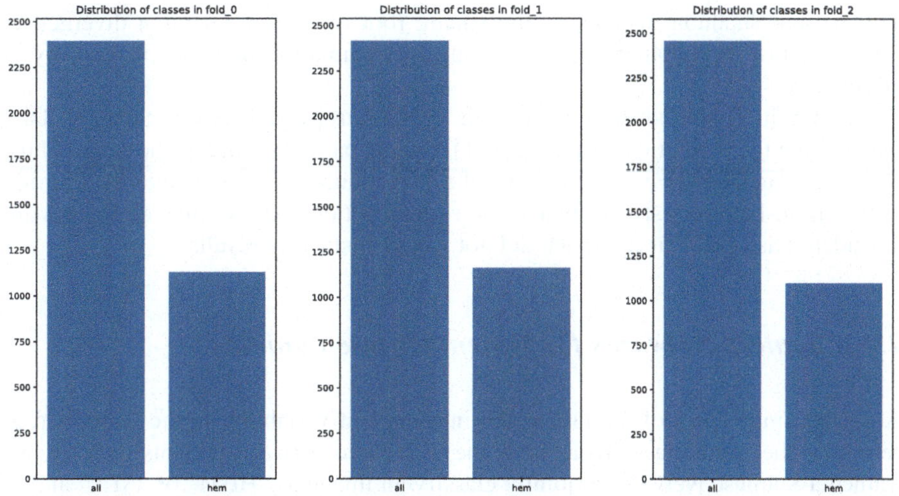

(a) Fold 0 Distribution (b) Fold 1 Distribution (c) Fold 2 Distribution

Fig. 1 Distribution of classes across folds

2.2 *Plain Feedforward Networks*

In the most naive approach, we fine-tuned the Inception V3 [10] and the ResNet50 [5] architectures (pretrained on the ImageNet dataset) on the training set. We observed that the weighted F1 on the validation set (0.85) was consistently less than that on the test set (0.90) for both the architectures for output sampled from different depths in the network.

2.3 *Optimizing Jensen–Shannon Distance*

In addition to the binary cross-entropy loss, we trained the network to minimize the Jensen–Shannon Distance as well. For n probability distributions (i.e., output class distributions of n samples in a batch), Jensen–Shannon divergence (JSD) is given as

$$JSD_{\pi_1,\ldots,\pi_n}(P_1, .., P_n) = H(\sum_{i=1}^{n} \pi_i P_i) - \sum_{i=1}^{n} \pi_i H(P_i) \tag{1}$$

where H is the Shannon Entropy given by

$$H(P) = -\sum_{k} P_{ik} \log(P_{ik}) \tag{2}$$

The Jensen–Shannon distance is the square root of Jensen–Shannon divergence. Since the task is of binary classification, the summation in Shannon Entropy is eliminated.

The intuition behind optimizing both, cross-entropy and Jensen–Shannon Distance is that the predictions for images of the same patient should be the same. Thus, we try to train the network to recognize the dependence between images. At training time, a mini-batch consists of images of a single patient. At test time, all images are considered as i.i.d. This approach did not yield satisfactory results.

2.4 Siamese Networks for Patient Differentiation

A challenging aspect of the task is the inter-patient variability in the features representing the same class. To address the difference between patients directly, we trained a Siamese Network to jointly classify an image as "HEM" or "ALL" and to differentiate between images of different patients. Details for the Siamese Network can be found in [18]. The final prediction vector of a Siamese Network is given as

$$p = \sigma(\sum_{j} \alpha_j \mid \mathbf{h}^{(j)}_{1,L-1} - \mathbf{h}^{(j)}_{2,L-1} \mid) \tag{3}$$

where $\mathbf{h}$ is the output of the penultimate layer. The prediction vector measures the similarity between the features calculated by the twins on two different images.

Intuitively, the cross-entropy loss for classification between 'HEM' and 'ALL' should force the network to learn features to distinguish between the classes. The cross-entropy loss for the Siamese Network should force the network to learn features that distinguish between different patients of the same class. Initial results on the validation data for this approach were not satisfactory, and due to time constraints, this approach was not taken forward.

3 i.i.d. Assumption

3.1 Data Preparation and Augmentation

By combining all the three folds and sampling images at random, we kept 70% of the total images for training, 15% for validation, and 15% for testing. The class distribution was maintained in each of the sets while splitting. We then augmented each class using the Augmentor [19] library so that we achieved a uniform distribution. Applied augmentations are described in Table 1. We have not used any online augmentation. We experimented with Inception V3 [10], DenseNet121 [7], ResNet50 [5], Xception [20], and ResNeXt [21] architectures. The results on the preliminary test set can be found in Table 3.

Table 1 Augmentations applied

Augmentation type	Probability	Other parameters (if any)
Flip horizontal	0.75	
Flip vertical	0.75	
Shear	0.4	max_shear_left = 4, max_shear_right = 4
Distortion	0.4	grid_width = 3, grid_height = 3, magnitude = 5
Zoom	0.4	min_factor = 1.1, max_factor = 1.5
Crop	0.5	Area = 0.8
Skew	0.3	Magnitude = 0.8

3.2 *Autoencoder-Based Approach*

We hypothesized that a Convolutional Autoencoder [22] might help us capture important information regarding each class, using which the classification task should become easier. We calculated the (per-pixel) means and standard deviations for each class separately and trained two custom convolutional autoencoders for the two classes in isolation. After a sufficiently optimum loss, we extracted the encoders, froze their weights, concatenated their latent representations, and stacked a Fully Connected network with a sigmoid activation at the end. However, this approach did not perform as per our expectations, because of which it was not taken forward.

3.3 *Ensemble of CNNs and Data Preprocessing*

We fine-tuned a total of 17 CNN architectures, of which the ResNeXt101 [21], DenseNet101 [7], and ResNet50 architectures were saved after training for two different durations. The images were preprocessed by architecture-specific preprocessing functions. The ResNeXt101, trained for a longer duration, achieved the highest online validation weighted F1 score of 0.8116. Following this, we fine-tuned four different models by placing the classification layer at different depths in the ResNeXt101 network, specifically at *conv4_block1*, *conv4_block8*, *conv4_block16*, and *conv4_block20*, saved after training for two different durations. Alongside the average ensemble, we also experimented with different meta-classifiers (neural nets, Random Forests, SVMs, etc.). Our highest score (0.825) for Phase I was achieved with the average ensemble of the two models cut at *conv4_block16*, the decision threshold of 0.4. The threshold was found after experimenting with various values ranging from 0.35 to 0.75.

Table 2 Online augmentation parameters

Augmentation type	Other parameters (if any)
Rotate	30° (CCW)
Horizontal flip	
Vertical flip	

4 Phase 2 Training

For the second phase of the competition, we used the entire training data given before as our training set and phase 1 labels as the hold-out data. Offline augmentation was skipped because we were of the opinion that the training data was sufficient enough to handle the imbalance. Online augmentation in the form of horizontal flip, vertical flip, and rotation was used. Distortion inducing transforms were not used to avoid inadvertent loss or change of features defining a class. The online augmentations performed are mentioned in Table 2.

Since the ResNeXt architecture was the best performer in Phase 1, it was chosen as the base architecture. After careful hyperparameter initialization, the final validation weighted F1 for the ResNeXt50 model was 0.857. We also trained a ResNeXt101 model, which converged at a final validation weighted F1 of 0.849.

4.1 Class Weights for Cost-Sensitive Training

An extensive study of the class imbalance problem in deep learning has been performed in [23]. Since a noticeable class imbalance is present, we use class weights while training. A misclassification of a minority class is assigned a higher loss than the majority class. The class weights are calculated as

$$W_c = \frac{n\_samples_t}{n\_classes * n\_samples_c} \tag{4}$$

where $n\_samples_t$ is the total number of images in the dataset, $n\_classes$ is the number of classes (in this case 2), and $n\_samples_c$ is the total number of images of class c [24].

It is to be noted that class weights are not used during inference time.

4.2 Augmentation Using GANs

In order to generate realistic images for the minority (HEM) class and combat class imbalance, we tried to generate synthetic data using the training data given. The obvious choice for doing so was to use Generative Adversarial Networks. We decided to go for two main subtypes of GANs—The W-GAN (Wasserstein GAN) [25] and the DCGAN (Deep Convolutional GAN) [26]. However, due to a shortage of time, this endeavor has been kept aside as a part of future scope.

5 Results

This section describes the results obtained on both the ResNeXt50 and ResNeXt101 architectures. For both the architectures, an initial learning rate of $7e^{-5}$ was used. The learning rate was decayed by 10% every three epochs. A batch decay of $5e^{-4}$ was also used. Both models were trained using the Adam [27] optimizer. Both models were trained for a total duration of 25 epochs. The Keras [28] framework was used to train both the models. Table 3 shows the results on the online preliminary test and test sets.

As can be seen from Fig. 2a, the validation loss for the ResNeXt101 model is very unstable despite using a very low learning rate. In comparison, the training loss smoothly decreases. This might be a symptom of overfitting. Figure 2b shows the weighted F1 plots for the ResNeXt101 model. The training F1 smoothly increases with respect to the number of epochs; however, the validation F1 behaves erratically.

Table 3 Weighted F1 score on preliminary test and test sets

Dataset	ResNeXt50	ResNeXt101	Inception V3	Xception	DenseNet121	ResNet50
Preliminary test	0.857	0.849	0.74	0.7305	0.7465	0.6245
Test	0.72	–	–	–	–	–

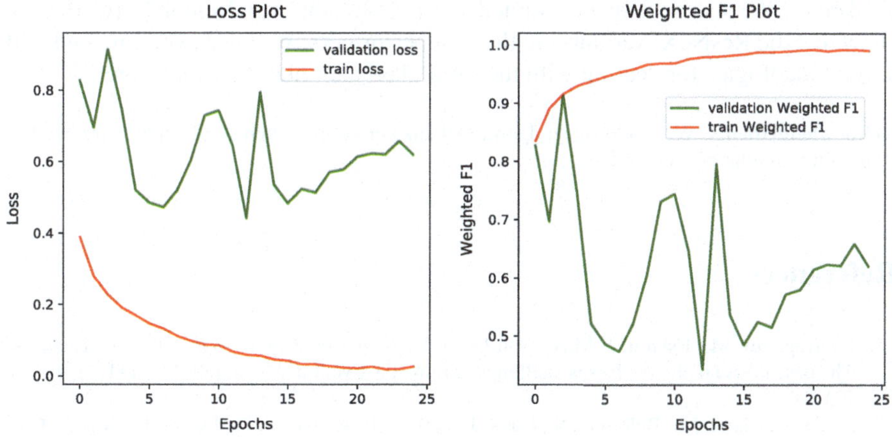

(a) ResNeXt101 Loss Plot (b) ResNeXt101 Weighted F1 Plot

Fig. 2 ResNeXt101 plots

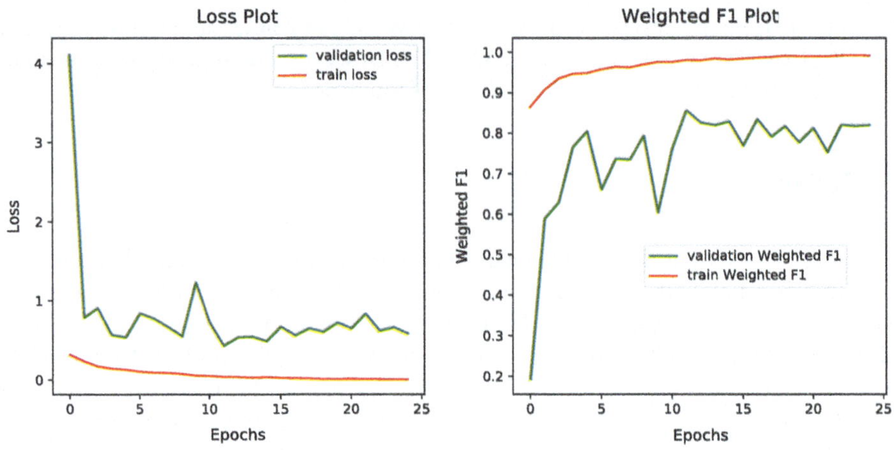

(a) ResNeXt50 Loss Plot (b) ResNeXt50 Weighted F1 Plot

Fig. 3 ResNeXt50 plots

In comparison, Fig. 3a shows that the loss plots for ResNeXt50 are much more controlled—the training loss decreases slowly, and the validation loss does not fluctuate too much. Figure 3b shows the weighted F1 plots for the ResNeXt50 model. This, too, shows indications of stable training.

6 Conclusion

We present a framework for the automated classification of B-Acute Lymphoblastic Leukemia. We use several pre-trained Deep Convolutional Neural Networks and show that the ResNeXt variants are the best performers. We have experimented with several ideologies for dealing with the intra-class and interclass variation.

Acknowledgements We would sincerely like to thank Persistent Systems Ltd. for their tremendous support throughout our research.

References

1. Everingham, M., Eslami, S.M.A., Van Gool, L., Williams, C.K.I., Winn, J., Zisserman, A.: The pascal visual object classes challenge: a retrospective. Int. J. Comput. Vis. **111**(1), 98–136 (2015)
2. Lin, T.Y., Maire, M., Belongie, S., Hays, J., Perona, P., Ramanan, D., Dollár, P., Zitnick, C.L.: Microsoft coco: common objects in context. In: Fleet, D., Pajdla, T., Schiele, B., Tuytelaars, T.

(eds.) Computer Vision—ECCV 2014, pp. 740–755. Springer International Publishing, Cham (2014)
3. Russakovsky, O., Deng, J., Su, H., Krause, J., Satheesh, S., Ma, S., Huang, Z., Karpathy, A., Khosla, A., Bernstein, M., Berg, A.C., Fei-Fei, L.: Imagenet large scale visual recognition challenge. Int. J. Comput. Vis. **115**(3), 211–252 (2015). https://doi.org/10.1007/s11263-015-0816-y
4. Krizhevsky, A., Sutskever, I., Hinton, G.E.: Imagenet classification with deep convolutional neural networks. In: Pereira, F., Burges, C.J.C., Bottou, L., Weinberger, K.Q. (eds.) Advances in Neural Information Processing Systems, vol. 25, pp. 1097–1105. Curran Associates, Inc. (2012). http://papers.nips.cc/paper/4824-imagenet-classification-with-deep-convolutional-neural-networks.pdf
5. He, K., Zhang, X., Ren, S., Sun, J.: Deep residual learning for image recognition. In: 2016 IEEE Conference on Computer Vision and Pattern Recognition (CVPR). pp. 770–778, June 2016. https://doi.org/10.1109/CVPR.2016.90
6. Hu, J., Shen, L., Sun, G.: Squeeze-and-excitation networks. In: The IEEE Conference on Computer Vision and Pattern Recognition (CVPR), June 2018
7. Huang, G., Liu, Z., v. d. Maaten, L., Weinberger, K.Q.: Densely connected convolutional networks. In: 2017 IEEE Conference on Computer Vision and Pattern Recognition (CVPR). pp. 2261–2269, July 2017. https://doi.org/10.1109/CVPR.2017.243
8. Simonyan, K., Zisserman, A.: Very deep convolutional networks for large-scale image recognition (2014). http://arxiv.org/abs/1409.1556
9. Szegedy, C., Sermanet, P., Reed, S., Anguelov, D., Erhan, D., Vanhoucke, V., Rabinovich, A.: Going deeper with convolutions. In: 2015 IEEE Conference on Computer Vision and Pattern Recognition (CVPR). pp. 1–9, June 2015. https://doi.org/10.1109/CVPR.2015.7298594
10. Szegedy, C., Vanhoucke, V., Ioffe, S., Shlens, J., Wojna, Z.: Rethinking the inception architecture for computer vision. In: 2016 IEEE Conference on Computer Vision and Pattern Recognition (CVPR). pp. 2818–2826, June 2016. https://doi.org/10.1109/CVPR.2016.308
11. Zeiler, M.D., Fergus, R.: Visualizing and understanding convolutional networks. In: Fleet, D., Pajdla, T., Schiele, B., Tuytelaars, T. (eds.) Computer Vision—ECCV 2014, pp. 818–833. Springer International Publishing, Cham (2014)
12. Ioffe, S., Szegedy, C.: Batch normalization: accelerating deep network training by reducing internal covariate shift. In: Bach, F., Blei, D. (eds.) Proceedings of the 32nd International Conference on Machine Learning. Proceedings of Machine Learning Research, vol. 37, pp. 448–456. PMLR, Lille, France, 07–09 July 2015. http://proceedings.mlr.press/v37/ioffe15.html
13. Gupta, A., Duggal, R., Gupta, R., Kumar, L., Thakkar, N., Satpathy, D.: GCTI-SN: Geometry-inspired chemical and tissue invariant stain normalization of microscopic medical images
14. Duggal, R., Gupta, A.G., Gupta, R.: Segmentation of overlapping/touching white blood cell nuclei using artificial neural networks. In: CME Series on Hemato-Oncopathology. All India Institute of Medical Sciences (AIIMS), New Delhi, India, July 2016
15. Duggal, R., Gupta, A., Gupta, R., Mallick, P.: Sd-layer: Stain deconvolutional layer for CNNs in medical microscopic imaging. In: Descoteaux M., Maier-Hein L., Franz A., Jannin P., Collins D., Duchesne S. (eds) Medical Image Computing and Computer-Assisted Intervention MICCAI 2017, MICCAI 2017. Lecture Notes in Computer Science, Part III, LNCS 10435, pp. 435–443. Springer, Cham, July 2016. https://doi.org/10.1007/978-3-319-66179-7_50
16. Duggal, R., Gupta, A., Gupta, R., Wadhwa, W., Ahuja, C.: Overlapping cell nuclei segmentation in microscopic images using deep belief networks. In: Indian Conference on Computer Vision, Graphics and Image Processing (ICVGIP), India, Dec 2016
17. Gupta, R., Mallick, P., Duggal, R., Gupta, A., Sharma, O.: Stain color normalization and segmentation of plasma cells in microscopic images as a prelude to development of computer assisted automated disease diagnostic tool in multiple myeloma. In: 16th International Myeloma Workshop (IMW), India, Mar 2017
18. Koch, G., Zemel, R., Salakhutdinov, R.: Siamese neural networks for one-shot image recognition. In: ICML Deep Learning Workshop (2015)

19. Bloice, M.D., Stocker, C., Holzinger, A.: Augmentor: an image augmentation library for machine learning (2017). http://arxiv.org/abs/1708.04680
20. Chollet, F.: Xception: Deep learning with depthwise separable convolutions. In: 2017 IEEE Conference on Computer Vision and Pattern Recognition (CVPR). pp. 1800–1807, July 2017. https://doi.org/10.1109/CVPR.2017.195
21. Xie, S., Girshick, R., Dollr, P., Tu, Z., He, K.: Aggregated residual transformations for deep neural networks. In: 2017 IEEE Conference on Computer Vision and Pattern Recognition (CVPR). pp. 5987–5995, July 2017. https://doi.org/10.1109/CVPR.2017.634
22. Masci, J., Meier, U., Cireşan, D., Schmidhuber, J.: Stacked convolutional auto-encoders for hierarchical feature extraction. In: Honkela, T., Duch, W., Girolami, M., Kaski, S. (eds.) Artificial Neural Networks and Machine Learning—ICANN 2011, pp. 52–59. Springer, Berlin Heidelberg, Berlin, Heidelberg (2011)
23. Buda, M., Maki, A., Mazurowski, M.A.: A systematic study of the class imbalance problem in convolutional neural networks (2017). http://arxiv.org/abs/1710.05381
24. Scikit learn class weights. https://goo.gl/Qwkxia
25. Arjovsky, M., Chintala, S., Bottou, L.: Wasserstein generative adversarial networks. In: Precup, D., Teh, Y.W. (eds.) Proceedings of the 34th International Conference on Machine Learning. Proceedings of Machine Learning Research, vol. 70, pp. 214–223. PMLR, International Convention Centre, Sydney, Australia, 06–11 Aug 2017. http://proceedings.mlr.press/v70/arjovsky17a.html
26. Radford, A., Metz, L., Chintala, S.: Unsupervised representation learning with deep convolutional generative adversarial networks (2015). arXiv preprint arXiv:1511.06434
27. Kingma, D.P., Ba, J.: Adam: A method for stochastic optimization (2014). arXiv preprint arXiv:1412.6980
28. Chollet, F., et al.: Keras (2015)

Neighborhood-Correction Algorithm for Classification of Normal and Malignant Cells

Yongsheng Pan, Mingxia Liu, Yong Xia and Dinggang Shen

Abstract Classification of normal and malignant cells observed under a microscope is an essential and challenging step in the development of a cost-effective computer-aided diagnosis tool for acute lymphoblastic leukemia. In this paper, we propose the neighborhood-correction algorithm (NCA) to address this challenge, which consists of three major steps, including (1) fine-tuning a pretrained residual network using training data and producing initial labels and feature maps for test data, (2) constructing a Fisher vector for each cell image based on its feature maps, and (3) correcting the initial label of each test cell image via the weighted majority voting based on its most similar neighbors. We have evaluated this algorithm on the database provided by the grand challenge on the classification of normal and malignant cells (C-NMC) in B-ALL white blood cancer microscopic images. Experimental results demonstrate that our proposed NCA achieves the weighted F1-score of 92.50% and balanced accuracy of 91.73% in the preliminary testing and achieves weighted F1-score of 91.04% in the final testing, which ranks the first in C-NMC. Associated code is available at https://github.com/YongshengPan/ISBI-NMC.

Keywords Microscopic image classification · Fisher vector · Residual network · Leukemia · B-lymphoblast cells

---

Y. Pan · Y. Xia (✉)
Research & Development Institute of Northwestern Polytechnical University, Shenzhen 518057, China
e-mail: yxia@nwpu.edu.cn

School of Computer Science and Engineering, Northwestern Polytechnical University, Xi'an 710072, China

Y. Pan · M. Liu · D. Shen (✉)
Department of Radiology and BRIC, University of North Carolina, Chapel Hill, NC 27599, USA
e-mail: dgshen@med.unc.edu

A. Gupta and R. Gupta (eds.), *ISBI 2019 C-NMC Challenge: Classification in Cancer Cell Imaging*, Lecture Notes in Bioengineering,
https://doi.org/10.1007/978-981-15-0798-4_8

1 Introduction

Acute lymphoblastic leukemia (ALL) is an acute cancer that affects millions of people globally, mostly children with age between 2 and 5 [15]. It is characterized by the development of plenty of immature lymphocytes in the bone marrow that interfere with the production of new blood cells. ALL is typically fatal within weeks or months if with less treatment and there is no reliable measure to prevent it. Thus, it is critical to perform early diagnosis to improve the survival rate.

Diagnosis of ALL is typically based on blood tests and bone marrow examination [5]. The mechanism involves that the genetic mutations result in rapid cell division and increased immature lymphocytes [10]. In advanced cancer stages, the cancer cells start growing in an unrestricted fashion, and therefore they are presented in much larger numbers as compared to the numbers in an early-stage patient. This could be identified by advanced methods such as flow cytometry [17], which, however, are too expensive to be widely used in less-developed regions.

As the morphology of cells can be observed under a microscope, it is possible to develop a cost-effective computer-aided solution to normal–malignant B-lymphoblast cell classification on microscopic images and hence to reduce the cost of ALL diagnosis. Recent years have witnessed the incredible advances in automated image classification [11, 12], including aggregative models [16] and deep convolutional neural networks (DCNNs) [12]. Since the image representation ability of DCNNs learned from large-scale datasets can be transferred to extract local descriptors on a generic image classification task, DCNNs have been combined with FV to boost the performance of image classification [1, 13, 14]. The Fisher vector (FV) and residual network (ResNet) [8] are typical representatives of aggregative models and DCNNs, respectively. The FV treats each image as a set of local visual descriptors sampled from a distribution under the label condition, and thus aggregates these descriptors into high-level image representations that can infer semantics and be separated linearly. The ResNet provides a uniform framework of feature extraction and classification to free users from the troublesome handcrafted feature extraction.

Despite these advances, it still remains a challenge to differentiate malignant cells from normal ones accurately since the morphological specificity of malignant cells appears very similar to that of normal cells [3, 4]. The grand challenge on classification of normal versus malignant cells (C-NMC) in B-ALL white blood cancer microscopic images organized in conjunction with the 2019 IEEE international symposium on biomedical imaging (ISBI 2019) recognized the significance and complexity of this image classification task and provided a database of clinical cells to evaluate various image classification approaches [7].

In this paper, we propose the neighborhood-correction algorithm (NCA) for the classification of normal–malignant B-lymphoblast cell images. To combine the advantages of ResNet and FV, we first fine-tune a pretrained ResNet (pRN) using training data and then use feature maps of each test image produced by the fine-tuned ResNet (fRN) as local descriptors to construct FVs. Finally, we correct the initial

Table 1 Distribution of C-NMC Challenge database

		Phase-I			Phase-II	Phase-III
		Fold 1	Fold 2	Fold 3		
Subjects	Cancer	19	11	17	13	9
	Normal	9	3	14	15	8
Cell images	Malignant	2397	2418	2457	1219	–
	Normal	1130	1163	1096	648	–

label predicted by fRN of each test cell image using the weighted majority voting based on its most similar neighbors. Our algorithm has been evaluated on the C-NMC Challenge database and achieved state-of-the-art performance.

2 Materials

The C-NMC Challenge database [7] contains the cell images from 84 cancer and 70 normal subjects, where the label of each cell is assumed to be the subject-level label. This dataset was released in three phases. 7272 malignant cells from 47 cancer subjects and 3389 normal cells from 26 normal subjects, together with a 3-fold data split, were released in Phase-I. 1219 malignant cells from 13 cancer subjects and 648 normal cells from 15 normal subjects were released in Phase-II. In Phase-III, the 2586 cell images from 9 cancer subjects and 8 normal subjects were released, but the label of each cell was withheld for online validation. The data distribution is illustrated in Table 1. All cells have been preprocessed via stain normalization and cell segmentation [2–4, 6, 7]. Each cell is roughly of size 300×300 and relocated at the center of a 450×450 baseplate.

3 Method

The proposed NCA mainly contains three steps. In Step 1, a pRN is fine-tuned using the training data to get the fRN, which can predict the initial labels and feature maps for test cells. In Step 2, the feature maps of each cell are aggregated to an FV, followed by calculating the dot product of FVs to measure the similarity of each pair of cells. In Step 3, the initial label of each cell is adjusted according to its neighborhood in the FV space. A diagram that summarizes our proposed model is shown in Fig. 1.

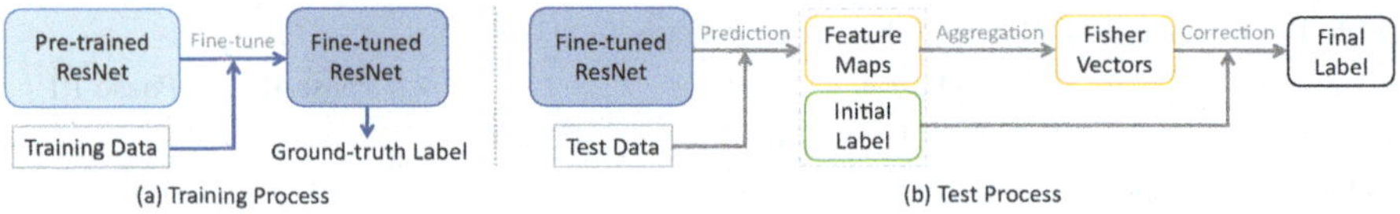

Fig. 1 Diagram of the proposed NCA algorithm for normal–malignant cell classification on microscopic images

3.1 Fine-Tuning ResNets

Since the C-NMC database is too small to train a DCNN with random initialization, we adopt the pRN, whose three off-the-shelf models (e.g., pRN50, pRN101, and pRN152) pretrained on the ImageNet database are available at the MatConvNet website [19], to avoid falling into overfitting when training. The architecture of a pRN contains a general convolutional layer followed with a max-pooling layer, dozens of residual blocks, and a fully connected layer. To apply the pRN to the normal–malignant cell classification, we keep only the first two neurons of the last fully connected layer and remove other neurons and related weights in this layer. While fine-tuning the pRN, each cell image is randomly rotated 0–350° for data augmentation and cropped to 224 × 224 to fit the input size in each of 20 epochs. The stochastic gradient descent (SGD) algorithm [18] is used as the optimizer with a batch size of 32 and a learning rate of 0.001 for the first 10 epochs and 0.0001 for the next 10 epochs. After obtaining the fRN, we rotate each test cell image 0–350° with an interval of 10°, thus resulting in 36 augmented copies, and then feed the cropped copies (size: 224 × 224) to fRN. The initial label of each test image is the majority voting result of its 36 augmented copies.

3.2 Combined ResNet-FV for Cell Representation

We extract the 7 × 7 × 512 feature maps produced by the "res5c_branch2a" layer of the fRN as local descriptors. Since each cell image has 36 augmented copies, we totally extract $N = 36 \times 7 \times 7$ descriptors, denoted as $X = \{x_n \in R^D; n = 1, \ldots, N\}$ $(D = 512)$. We assume that these descriptors of all cell images follow a Gaussian mixture model (GMM) u_θ with diagonal covariance, whose parameters $\theta = \{\omega_l, \mu_l, \sigma_l; l = 1, \ldots, L\}$ are estimated by the maximum likelihood estimation (MLE). Then, the FV of X is defined as the Fisher information normalized gradient of the log likelihood [7] of X with respect to each mean μ_l and standard deviation σ_l, shown as follows:

$$\mathcal{B}_\theta = (\mathcal{B}_{\mu,1}{}^{\mathrm{T}}, \ldots, \mathcal{B}_{\mu,L}{}^{\mathrm{T}}, \mathcal{B}_{\sigma,1}{}^{\mathrm{T}}, \ldots, \mathcal{B}_{\sigma,L}{}^{\mathrm{T}})^{\mathrm{T}}, \tag{1}$$

where

$$\begin{cases} \mathcal{B}_{l,\mu} = \frac{1}{N\sqrt{\omega_l}} \sum_{n=1}^{N} \tau_l(x_n) \left[\frac{x_n - \mu_l}{\sigma_l} \right], \\ \mathcal{B}_{l,\sigma} = \frac{1}{N\sqrt{2\omega_l}} \sum_{n=1}^{N} \tau_l(x_n) \left[\frac{(x_n - \mu_l)^2}{\sigma_l^2} - 1 \right], \end{cases} \tag{2}$$

and $\tau_l(x_n) = \frac{\omega_l \mu_l(x_n)}{\sum_{j=1}^{L}[\omega_j u_j(x_n)]}$ is the posterior probability of x_n being assigned to the lth Gaussian component u_l. To cancel out the effect that cells at different grades of maturity may have different sizes and thus result in biased FV signatures, the following l_2-normalization [16] is then employed

$$\mathfrak{B}_\theta^X = \mathcal{B}_\theta^X / \left\| \mathcal{B}_\theta^X \right\|_2 \tag{3}$$

The Fisher kernel (FK) that measures the similarity between two cell images X_1 and X_2 is defined as

$$J_{FK}(X_1, X_2) = \mathfrak{B}_\theta^{X_1\,\mathrm{T}} \mathfrak{B}_\theta^{X_2} \tag{4}$$

Incidentally, this kernel can be cooperated with a support vector machine (SVM) [1] for cell image classification.

3.3 Label Correction

After obtaining the FV and initial label of each testing cell image, we can use the neighborhood information to correct misclassified images. We assume that the images with similar discriminative representations (i.e., FVs) belong to the same category. Suppose that $X_{i,(1)}, X_{i,(2)}, \ldots, X_{i,(K)}$ are the most similar K images of X_i, whose initial labels are $y_{i,(1)}, y_{i,(2)}, \ldots, y_{i,(K)}$, respectively, where $X_{i,(1)} = X_i$ and $y_{i,(1)} = y_i$ since the most similar image is itself. If the label of X_i is different from any of its K nearest neighbors in the FV space, we adjust the label of X_i as the weighted voting result of $y_{i,(1)}, \ldots, y_{i,(K)}$ as follows:

$$y_i^* = \text{sign}\left[\sum_{k=1}^{K} J(X_i, X_{i,(k)}) y_{i,(K)} \right] \tag{5}$$

where $J(X_1, X_2)$ equals $J_{FK}(X_1, X_2)$ if only one fRN is used, or the minimum of J_{FK} values if multiple fRNs are used.

4 Experiments and Discussions

We performed three groups of experiments to evaluate our NCA on the C-NMC database. We first evaluated the impact of different ResNets, and then compared NCA to three methods on the Phase-I dataset. We finally applied NCA to the Phase-II dataset. We set $L = 8$ in the aggregative model and $K = 7$ for label correction. The accuracy of each method is measured by the weighted F1-score (WF1S) and the balanced accuracy (BACC) [9].

4.1 Cross-Validation of Baseline Method

We first evaluated the baseline method (BM) that directly applied fRN to test data via 3-fold cross-validation. Each time, one of the three folds was used to test the fRN fine-tuned on the other two folds. The WF1S and BACC values achieved by BM (including fRN50, fRN101, and fRN152) were shown in Fig. 2, where the horizontal axis indicates the performance on each of the three folds and the average (AVG) performance. Figure 2 reveals that (1) fRN101 results in slightly higher average WF1S and BACC values than fRN50 and fRN152, (2) no matter which fRN was used, using Fold-0 and Fold-2 as the test dataset leads to the highest and lowest accuracy, respectively, largely due to the inconsistency over subjects, and (3) the performance variation caused by different fRNs is much less than that caused by different test datasets.

4.2 Performance Gain Caused by Label Correction

In the second group of experiments, we evaluated the effectiveness of our NCA by comparing it to BM and FV with the linear SVM as the classifier. Herein, Res-Net-50 (with 50 layers) was used for all methods. For FV, we considered both the FV with

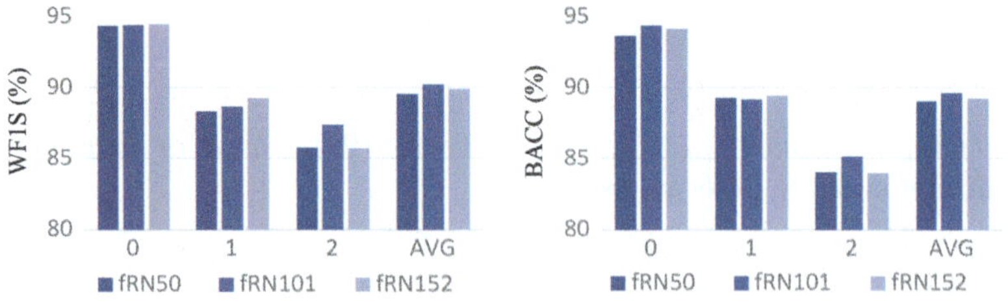

Fig. 2 WF1S (left) and BACC (right) values (%) obtained by fRN50/101/152 in 3-fold cross-validation. The horizontal axis indicates the result on Fold-0/1/2 and the average result

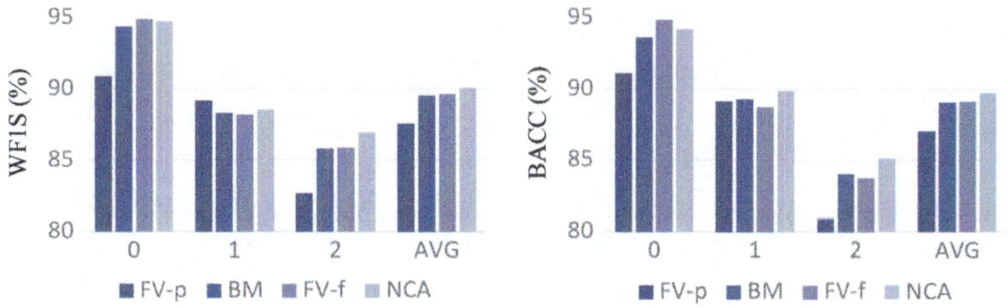

Fig. 3 WF1S (left) and BACC (right) values (%) obtained by four methods based on ResNet-50, where NCA produces the highest metrics on average (AVG)

the pRN50 (FV-p) and the FV with fRN50 (FV-f). The WF1S and BACC values for three folds and their average are shown in Fig. 3. From Fig. 3, we can see that NCA generally outperforms three competing methods regarding the average values of both metrics. Meanwhile, FV-f and NCA perform the best on Fold-0 and Fold-2, respectively while NCA and FV-p reach the best WF1S and BACC on Fold-1, respectively. Compared to BM, the improved BACC/WF1S values of NCA are 0.59/0.39%, 0.59/0.24%, and 1.09/1.15% for Fold-0, Fold-1, and Fold-2, respectively. All these results indicate that our NCA is successful in C-NMC and is useful for ALL diagnosis. Besides, BM, FV-f, and NCA are superior to FV-p obviously while FV-f reaches a comparable but slightly better performance than BM. It indicates that the fine-tuned pRN model can increase the distinguishability for cell representation and the FK is good at measuring the similarity of cells. Therefore, it is reasonable to use FV with fRN to estimate the data distribution of cell images. Particularly, our NCA achieves the largest improvement on Fold-2, on which the other three methods achieve the worst metrics. This suggests that our NCA may have an outstanding capability to boost the unsatisfying performance.

4.3 *Results on Phase-II Dataset*

In the third group of experiments, we used the Phase-II dataset to further evaluate our NCA against BM. We considered different combinations that use one, two, or three folds in Phase-I for training, with Phase-II used for external validation. The BACC and WF1S values are reported in Table 2. While using single fold for training, the models trained on Fold-1 perform much worse than those trained on Fold-0 or Fold-2, almost no better than random guesses. The reason lies in the fact that Fold-1 contains only three normal subjects, which results in a large negative bias to the trained models. While using two folds for training, the models trained on Fold-0 and Fold-1 perform much worse than those on Fold-0 and Fold-2 and those on Fold-1 and Fold-2. This again verifies that the cells among different folds (or different subjects) are inconsistent, which is attributed mainly to the heterogeneous data acquisition process. Also, the models trained on all three folds perform obviously better than the

Table 2 WF1S/BACC of 21 pairs of comparisons on Phase-II (%)

Fold			Method	ResNet-50		ResNet-101		ResNet-152	
0	1	2		WF1S	BACC	WF1S	BACC	WF1S	BACC
✓			BM	78.54	78.23	78.78	79.01	77.37	76.68
			NCA	**81.42**	**81.89**	**82.87**	**83.77**	**79.25**	**79.07**
	✓		BM	**52.88**	**56.46**	**48.52**	**53.91**	**52.53**	**56.00**
			NCA	50.62	55.24	44.72	52.46	49.08	54.13
		✓	BM	76.70	78.95	80.32	82.28	76.65	78.39
			NCA	**77.40**	**80.22**	**80.98**	**83.27**	**77.67**	**80.33**
✓	✓		BM	67.82	66.80	70.30	68.92	72.46	70.98
			NCA	**72.90**	**71.32**	**73.81**	**72.00**	**76.00**	**74.19**
✓		✓	BM	83.55	84.41	83.55	84.27	80.60	81.27
			NCA	**84.32**	**85.93**	**84.21**	**85.67**	**82.04**	**83.39**
	✓	✓	BM	84.01	83.35	82.79	82.34	81.32	80.27
			NCA	**88.11**	**87.89**	**84.37**	**84.19**	**85.41**	**84.38**
✓	✓	✓	BM	83.69	83.00	84.27	84.11	84.11	83.64
			NCA	**88.41**	**87.99**	**85.51**	**85.92**	**85.41**	**85.88**

average of those models trained on one or two folds and are even similar to the best models trained on two folds. This indicates that using more data will further improve the performance.

Except for the results on only Fold-1, our NCA consistently outperforms BM on both metrics; even the increments are different on different fold combinations and different ResNets. When all three folds are used, the average results of BM and NCA over three ResNets are 84.02/83.58% and 86.44/86.60%, respectively, achieving an increment of 2.42/3.02%. Particularly, NCA achieves the best result of 88.41/87.99% on ResNet-50. Using the ensemble of fRN50, fRN101, and fRN152, NCA achieves 92.50% and 91.73% of WF1S and BACC, respectively, which achieves the top result on the leaderboard of preliminary testing. NCA also ranks the first (91.04% of WF1S) in the final testing (Phase-III) while using data in both Phase-I and Phase-II to fine-tune ResNets.

4.4 Feedback to BM

In the third group of experiments, we have corrected the initial labels of cell images in Phase-II with obtaining fRNs on Phase-I and those in Phase-III with obtaining fRNs on Phase-I and Phase-II. Actually, these cell images with corrected labels can be further cooperated with these cell images with real labels to improve the BM. For example, we can improve the BM by fine-tuning the pRN-50 with both the cells with a real label in Phase-I and the cells with a corrected label in Phase-II. The performance

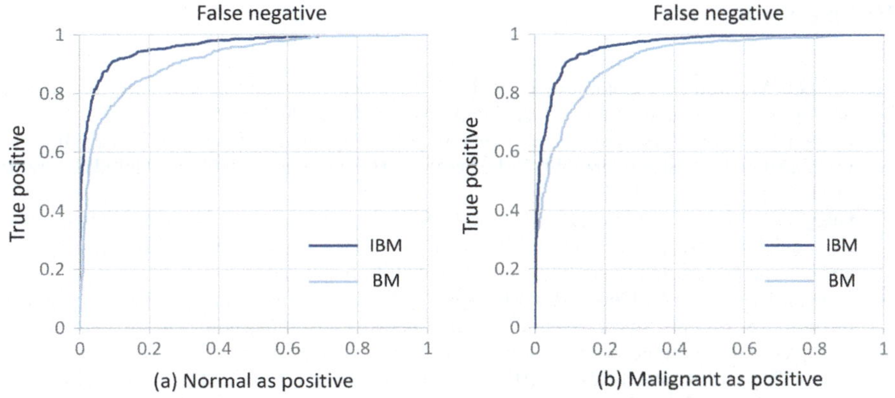

Fig. 4 WF1S (left) and BACC (right) values (%) obtained by four methods based on ResNet-50, where NCA produces the highest metrics on average (AVG)

curves of BM and the improved BM (IBM) are illustrated in Fig. 4, where Fig. 4a is the case considering normal cells as positive and Fig. 4b is the case considering malignant cells as positive. It can be seen that in both cases, IBM outperforms BM obviously. The area under the curve (AUC) is 91.52%, and 96.14% for BM and IBM, respectively, which indicates a huge improvement of 4.62%.

5 Conclusion

We have developed a neighborhood-correction algorithm (NCA) for normal–malignant cell classification on microscopic images. Results on the C-NMC database show that the NCA achieved acceptable accuracy on cell image classification. Our future work will focus on developing a unified framework for feature learning and label correction.

Acknowledgements Y. Pan and Y. Xia were supported in part by the Science and Technology Innovation Committee of Shenzhen Municipality, China, under Grants JCYJ20180306171334997, in part by the National Natural Science Foundation of China under Grants 61771397, in part by the Innovation Foundation for Doctor Dissertation of Northwestern Polytechnical University under Grants CX201835, and in part by the Project for Graduate Innovation team of Northwestern Polytechnical University.

References

1. Cimpoi, M., Maji, S., Kokkinos, I., Vedaldi, A.: Deep filter banks for texture recognition, description, and segmentation. Int. J. Comput. Vis. **118**(1), 65–94 (2016)
2. Duggal, R., Gupta, A., Gupta, R.: Segmentation of overlapping/touching white blood cell nuclei using artificial neural networks. In: CME Series on Hemato-Oncopathology. All India Institute of Medical Sciences (AIIMS) (2016)
3. Duggal, R., Gupta, A., Gupta, R., Mallick, P.: SD-layer: stain deconvolutional layer for CNNs in medical microscopic imaging. In: International Conference on Medical Image Computing and Computer-Assisted Intervention, pp. 435–443. Springer (2017)
4. Duggal, R., Gupta, A., Gupta, R., Wadhwa, M., Ahuja, C.: Overlapping cell nuclei segmentation in microscopic images using deep belief networks. In: Proceedings of the Tenth Indian Conference on Computer Vision, Graphics and Image Processing, p. 82. ACM (2016)
5. Ferri, F.F.: Ferri's Clinical Advisor 2018 E-Book: 5 Books in 1. Elsevier Health Sciences (2017)
6. Gupta, A., Duggal, R., Gupta, R., Kumar, L., Thakkar, N., Satpathy, D.: GCTI-SN: geometry-inspired chemical and tissue invariant stain normalization of microscopic medical images (under review)
7. Gupta, R., Mallick, P., Duggal, R., Gupta, A., Sharma, O.: Stain color normalization and segmentation of plasma cells in microscopic images as a prelude to development of computer assisted automated disease diagnostic tool in multiple myeloma. Clin. Lymphoma Myeloma Leukemia **17**(1), e99 (2017)
8. He, K., Zhang, X., Ren, S., Sun, J.: Deep residual learning for image recognition. In: Proceedings of the IEEE Conference on Computer Vision and Pattern Recognition, pp. 770–778 (2016)
9. Hripcsak, G., Rothschild, A.S.: Agreement, the F-measure, and reliability in information retrieval. J. Am. Med. Inform. Assoc. **12**(3), 296–298 (2005)
10. Hunger, S.P., Mullighan, C.G.: Acute lymphoblastic leukemia in children. New Engl. J. Med. **373**(16), 1541–1552 (2015)
11. Li, Z., Song, Y., Mcloughlin, I., Dai, L.: Compact convolutional neural network transfer learning for small-scale image classification. In: 2016 IEEE International Conference on Acoustics, Speech and Signal Processing (ICASSP), pp. 2737–2741. IEEE (2016)
12. Lin, T.Y., RoyChowdhury, A., Maji, S.: Bilinear convolutional neural networks for fine-grained visual recognition. IEEE Trans. Pattern Anal. Mach. Intell. **40**(6), 1309–1322 (2018)
13. Liu, L., Wang, P., Shen, C., Wang, L., Van Den Hengel, A., Wang, C., Shen, H.T.: Compositional model based Fisher vector coding for image classification. IEEE Trans. Pattern Anal. Mach. Intell. **39**(12), 2335–2348 (2017)
14. Pan, Y., Xia, Y., Shen, D.: Foreground Fisher Vector: Encoding Class-Relevant Foreground to Improve Image Classification. IEEE (accepted on 2019)
15. Pui, C.H.: Acute Lymphoblastic Leukemia. Springer (2011)
16. Sánchez, J., Perronnin, F., Mensink, T., Verbeek, J.: Image classification with the Fisher vector: theory and practice. Int. J. Comput. Vis. **105**(3), 222–245 (2013)
17. Shapiro, H.M.: Practical Flow Cytometry. Wiley (2005)
18. Teng, M., Wood, F.: Bayesian distributed stochastic gradient descent. In: Advances in Neural Information Processing Systems, pp. 6380–6390 (2018)
19. Vedaldi, A., Lenc, K.: Matconvnet: convolutional neural networks for MATLAB. In: Proceedings of the 23rd ACM International Conference on Multimedia, pp. 689–692. ACM (2015)

DeepMEN: Multi-model Ensemble Network for B-Lymphoblast Cell Classification

Fenrui Xiao, Ruifeng Kuang, Zhonghong Ou and Baiqiao Xiong

Abstract In recent years, convolutional neural networks have achieved great results in many image classification tasks, including the field of medical image processing. However, for leukemic B-lymphoblast cells, the traditional convolutional neural network has some problems. On the one hand, there is a strong individual difference in the cell image, that is, there is a big difference between the cells of different subjects, and this difference may exceed the difference between abnormal cells and normal cells. On the other hand, the two cell types appear very similar. People without expertise can't tell if a cell is abnormal. In order to solve the above problems, we proposed Deep Multi-model Ensemble Network (DeepMEN). We trained a series of deep learning models and selected the six models with the most potential as candidates. We trained the six models respectively and used the model ensemble technology to fuse the six models. In addition, we use the pseudo-label and Test Time Augmentator (TTA) to reduce covariance shifts caused by individual differences. Finally, we obtained a weighted F1-score of 0.903 in the preliminary test set and 0.8856 in the final test set.

Keywords Deep learning · Covariance shift · Model ensemble

Fenrui Xiao and Ruifeng Kuang—The two authors contributed equally to this work.

F. Xiao (✉) · R. Kuang · Z. Ou · B. Xiong
Beijing University of Posts and Telecommunications, Beijing, China
e-mail: xiaofenrui@bupt.edu.cn

R. Kuang
e-mail: kuangruifeng@bupt.edu.cn

Z. Ou
e-mail: Zhonghong.ou@bupt.edu.cn

B. Xiong
e-mail: bq.Xiong@bupt.edu.cn

A. Gupta and R. Gupta (eds.), *ISBI 2019 C-NMC Challenge: Classification in Cancer Cell Imaging*, Lecture Notes in Bioengineering,
https://doi.org/10.1007/978-981-15-0798-4_9

1 Introduction

In recent years, convolutional neural networks [1, 2] have achieved great success in medical image recognition, and have been widely used in many aspects, such as blood vessel segmentation [3], lung nodule detection [4], blood cell classification [5], etc. Deep convolutional neural networks usually extract low/mid/high-level features [6] and classify images by classifier. By stacking convolutional layers, deep convolutional neural networks can obtain rich and different levels of information.

However, although deep convolutional neural networks have achieved good results on many tasks, the mainstream deep convolutional neural network cannot achieve the best performance for the leukemic B-lymphoblast cells. As shown in the Fig. 1, there is a big difference between the B-lymphoblast cells and the image in the ImageNet [7], which is the most commonly used classification dataset. The images in ImageNet contain more high-level semantics such as person and bike, while the B-lymphoblast cell images are more low-level semantic information such as texture information.

On the other hand, abnormal and healthy B-lymphoblast cells are very similar in cell morphology. As shown in the Fig. 2, people without professional knowledge cannot tell which cells are diseased. In addition, in our experiment, we found that there were strong individual differences in B-lymphoblast cells sampled from different patients, which led to the difficulty in maintaining consistent distribution of training set and test set. Moreover, training deep convolutional neural networks requires a large amount of annotated data, so that the trained model has the best generalization performance without over-fitting the training set. But in medical images, data shortage is a serious problem. Therefore, it is very challenging to ensure that the model has good generalization performance.

In order to solve the above problems, we have done a lot of work. Firstly, we use the method of the model ensemble to comprehensively utilize the feature extraction ability of different models and obtain better feature representation and results. In the first place, we tried a series of image classification models and tested their performance on the validation set. Then we selected six models that perform well. These models are trained separately on the training set to obtain the best performance

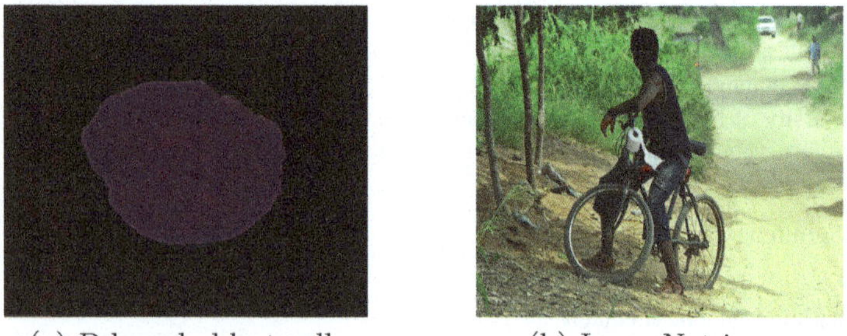

(a) B-lymphoblast cell (b) ImageNet image

Fig. 1 Images from B-lymphoblast cell and ImageNet

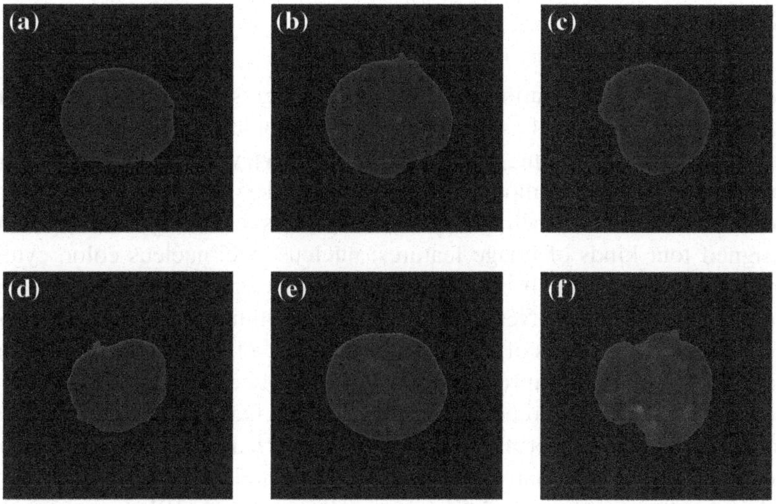

Fig. 2 Some B-lymphoblast cell images. **a–c** are abnormal and **d–f** are normal. We can see that they are very similar and there are no obvious features to distinguish them

model. In the end, we average the output probabilities of the six models and obtain the final prediction results based on this probability with the threshold 0.5. Model ensemble fully take the advantages of different models in different dimensions, which can reduce the variance and avoids overffiting effectively.

Secondly, in order to solve the problem of inconsistent distribution between the training set and test set, we use pseudo-label [8], a semi-supervised learning method, which uses the model trained by the training set to annotate the test set, obtaining the test set with the pseudo-label. The test set is added to the training set, and the whole model is trained again with the training set and test set with pseudo-label. After several iterations, the model is able to optimize the decision boundaries and continually learn and improve performance on the test set. This method can effectively improve the generalization ability of the model in the test set.

Finally, we used TTA technology to achieve more stable predicted results. TTA is simply to apply different transformations to test images like rotations, flipping, and translations. Then feed these different transformed images to the trained model and average the results to get a more confident answer. In our method, we use six transformations to test images and observe stable one percent improvement on the all single model.

In summary, we have done the following works: (1) We ensemble multiple deep learning models, which makes better predictions. (2) We use the pseudo-label method to enhance the generalization ability of the model (3) We use the TTA to get more confident predicts. Based on the above work, we finally achieved 0.8856 F1-score in the ISBI2019 CNMC[1] challenge final test set.

[1]Classification of Normal versus Malignant Cells in B-ALL White Blood Cancer Microscopic Images: ISBI 2019.

2 Related Work

The key to the cell classification algorithm is the expression of cell image features. Previously related cell classification features mainly include handcraft features, fisher vector, and dictionary learning, etc. We will briefly review and discuss in this section.

Early cell classification models often use hand-designed features and combine with traditional classifiers such as Bayesian classifiers to classify cell images. Young [9] designed four kinds of image features: nucleus size, nucleus color, cytoplasm size, and cytoplasm color. It classified 199 cells based on such four-dimensional feature space with KNN (k-Nearest Neighbor) algorithm; Fisher vector is a method for encoding global features of images, [10] presents a fisher tensor that can encode additional information to improve the performance of cell classification; Dictionary learning can extract sparse representations of image features, making the classifier more discriminating. Kong et al. [11] uses a dictionary learning algorithm to construct a more robust and discriminative cell classification model.

In the past few years, convolutional neural networks [12] have achieved great success in medical image recognition. Bayramoglu et al. [13] discuss the method of regularization, preprocessing, and image enhancement of Hep-2 cell images. It was proved that the selection of appropriate image preprocessing methods can significantly improve the classification effect of immunofluorescence images. Lei et al. [14] proposed a deep learning network based on ResNet50 to improve the classification effect of HEp-2 cells, combined with cross-modal transfer learning, which enhanced the generalization ability of the model and proved the deep learning method can be used to solve human cell classification problems. Xue and Ray [15] use output coding based on deep learning to improve the accuracy of microscopic cell detection. Duggal et al. [16] propose SD-Layer which can converts the original image into the optical density space, and combined with CNN to classify cell images, which achieved better performance on several basic CNN structures.

To sum up, the traditional image classification algorithm has made some achievements. However, there are still some problems such as weak feature expression ability, which makes it difficult to solve complex medical image processing problems. A deep convolutional neural network, as a tool with strong feature expression ability has made rich achievements in the field of medical image processing. Therefore, we choose to use the method of deep learning to deal with the classification of B-lymphocytes, and more detailed information will be introduced in the Sect. 3.

3 Methodology

3.1 Network Architecture

Since deep learning has been successful in many fields, we first tested the classification effect on the mainstream deep convolutional neural network architecture, as

Table 1 Model performance

Model	Precision	Recall	F1-score
AlexNet [2]	0.745	0.723	0.675
DenseNet121 [20]	0.874	0.874	**0.874**
DenseNet161 [20]	0.877	0.871	0.873
ResNet50	0.825	0.823	0.815
ResNet101	0.871	0.872	**0.870**
Dpn68 [21]	0.720	0.718	0.680
Dpn107 [21]	0.769	0.768	0.768
SENet154 [22]	0.871	0.873	**0.871**
SEResNext101	0.851	0.852	0.848
VGG16	0.877	0.878	**0.877**
DeepTEN	0.872	0.873	**0.871**
Inceptionv4 [23]	0.864	0.862	**0.863**
DeepMEN	**0.904**	**0.905**	**0.903**

shown in Table 1.[2] As can be seen from the table, the performance of ResNet101 [17] is better than that of ResNet50 [17], which indicates that increasing the depth of the network can improve the effectiveness of models. But that doesn't mean the deeper, the better. Shallow convolutional neural networks such as VGG16 [18] have achieved the highest score of 0.877. The shallow network retains more information about the underlying details, which is of great significance for the recognition of cell texture. In addition, we also tried to use texture classification method to deal with cell classification. DeepTEN [19] is a kind of texture coding network, which promotes the traditional dictionary learning and residual Encoding, and is compatible with deep learning constructs, achieving F1-score 0.871.

We select six models with the results from the Table 1 for model ensemble, which are DenseNet121, ResNet101, SENet154, VGG16, DeepTEN, and InceptionV4, respectively. We take an average of predictions from all the models and use them to make the final prediction. We first trained six models on the training set and get the best results. After that, each model was used to independently predict the test set and obtain the predicted probability. Then, the sum of the probability values was averaged as the final prediction result, and 0.5 was used as the threshold to obtain the predicted classification. Finally, the 0.903 F1-score was achieved with the model ensemble.

The final structure of our method is shown in the Fig. 3, which is an iterative approach. First, each model is trained using only the training set data and obtain six optimal models. After that, the model ensemble is carried out to obtain the final predictions. The prediction result is used to label the test set and get the pseudo-label

[2]Since the label of the final test set cannot be obtained, all the following experimental results are completed based on the preliminary test set.

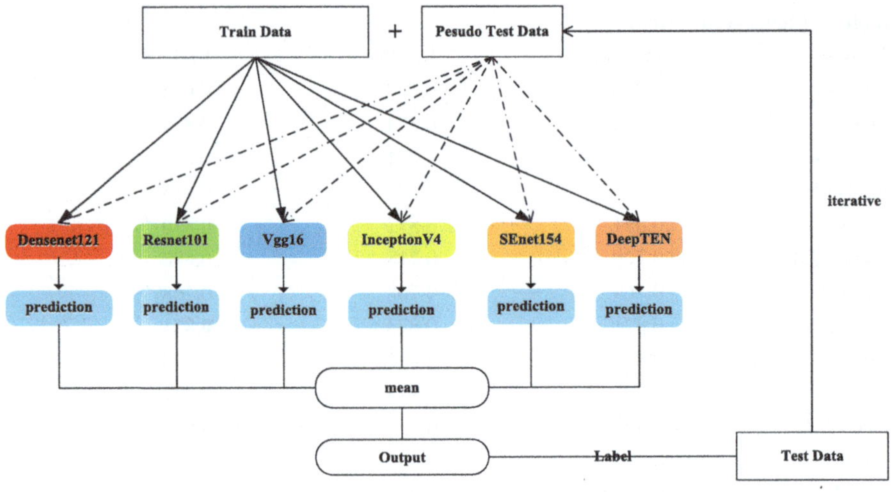

Fig. 3 The architecture of DeepMEN

about the test set. The test set data with pseudo-labels were added into the training set. Train the models again and a better prediction result was obtained after the same process. The final prediction result will be constantly optimized through iteration. About pseudo-label, we will introduce in detail in the following section.

3.2 Pseudo Labeling

Pseudo Labeling is a technique applying semi-supervised learning which is aimed to improve the generalization ability using unlabeled data. In this technique, instead of manually labeling the unlabeled data, we can get approximate labels based on the labeled data. Figure 3 illustrates the procedure of our method that how we apply Pseudo Labeling to improve the performance of our model. First, the network is trained in a supervised fashion with labeled data. As for unlabeled data, Pseudo-Labels are referred from pretrained network by picking up the class has the maximum predicted probability. Then the network is retrained with labeled data and pseudo-labeled data as if they were ground truth. Pseudo Labeling usually use pseudo-labels only once, but to increase our test score we update pseudo-labeled data iteratively because everytime we add pseudo-labeled data to training set we get more ground truth data.

3.3 Test Time Augmentor

TTA is simply to apply different transformations to test image like: rotations, flipping, and translations. Then feed these different transformed images to the trained model and average the results to get a more confident answer. In our method, we use six transformations to test image including rotation of 30°, 60°, 90°, and 180°, filp up and down. With TTA, our final result was improved from 0.903 to 0.905 in the preliminary test set, and 0.8856 in the final test set.

3.4 Training Details

All the models were trained using stochastic gradient descent (SGD). The initial learning rate was set to 0.003. Cosine annealing was used to schedule learning rate. The learning rate is calculated with the following formula:

$$LR = baseLR * 0.5 * (1 + \cos(\pi * Iter/maxIter)) \quad (1)$$

where $baseLR$ is the base learning rate set at the beginning, $Iter$ is the number of current iteration, and $maxIter$ is the number of iterations which is defined as following:

$$maxIter = epoch * itersPerEpoch \quad (2)$$

where $epoch$ is the number of current epoch, $itersPerEpoch$ is the number of iterations per epoch.

The batch size, momentum, and weight decay were set to 32, 0.9 and 0.001 for the training phase.

4 Experiment

Our data come from the ISBI2019 Challenge [16, 24, 25], and this section will provide a brief introduction to the dataset and the preprocessing methods we use.

4.1 Datasets

Our dataset contains a total of 118 independent subjects, of which 69 are cancerous subjects and 49 are normal subjects, which are divided into train set, preliminary test set, and final test set. The train set contains 76 subjects, of which 47 are abnormal and 29 are normal. There is a total of 10,661 cells, of which 7272 are abnormal cells and 3389 are normal cells. The preliminary test set contains 30 subjects, with 15 normal subjects and 15 abnormal subjects and the final test set contains 17 subjects, with 8 normal subjects and 9 abnormal subjects.

4.2 Image Preprocessing

We first center crop original image by removing the extra black edges and retaining only the cellular texture content. The size of the cropped image is 224×224. We did not take any resize operation to avoid damaging the texture. Then we normalize the image with the image mean and variance, constraining the input to the range $[-1, 1]$. Image enhancement is a very common method to enhance data. We have tried a series of image enhancement algorithms, such as enhanced contrast, and superpixels, but did not achieve the desired effect. We guess that image enhancement destroys the original texture information of cells and introduces new noise which makes the model more difficult to train and thus affects the final performance. Therefore, we ended up using only random rotations, up-down inversions, and random filp for image enhancement.

4.3 Result

We do some experiments to evaluate our model. We compare the model with the current mainstream convolutional neural network and all models were trained on 10,661 cell images and tested on a validation set containing 1867 images. We obtain the result and which is shown in Table 1. Our model achieved 90.4% accuracy, 90.5% recall, and 0.903 F1-score. By adjusting the final decision threshold from 0.5 to 0.525, we finally obtained F1-score 0.907.

Figure 4 shows the change of accuracy in positive samples, negative samples, and all samples with the change of threshold. It can be seen that our model does not fluctuate significantly with the change of threshold value indicating that our prediction results have a high degree of confidence and our model is very reliable.

Figure 5 shows the subject level accuracy in the preliminary test set. As can be seen from the figure, the model has achieved good results for most subjects, but for a small number of samples, the performance of the model is not ideal, indicating that the model's generalization ability has space for further improvement.

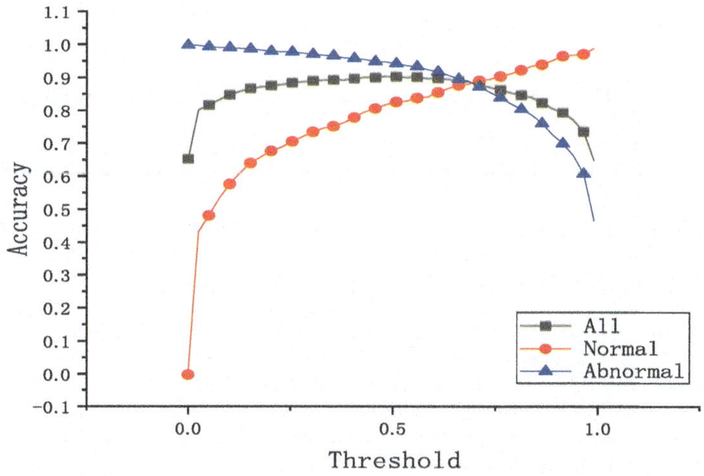

Fig. 4 Accuracy graph

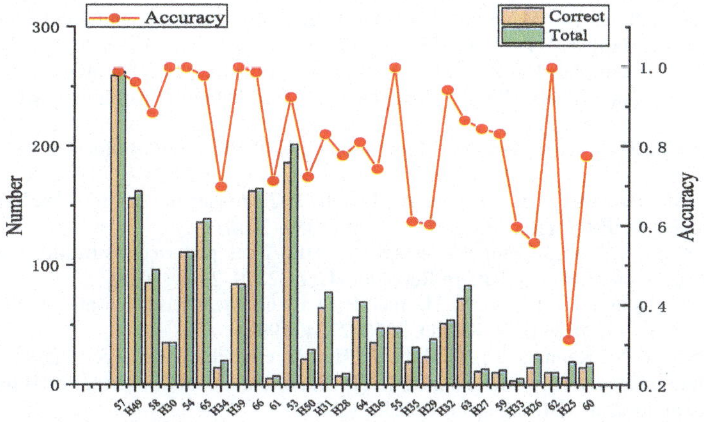

Fig. 5 Subject level accuracy graph

5 Conclusion

This paper proposed an effective B-lymphoblast cell classification pipeline. In the preprocessing phase, the most important cell regions were retained using central cropping and simple image enhancements without destroying the cell texture. In terms of model, six depth models are used for fusion to fully extract image features. During the prediction phase, TTA was used to make the prediction results more stable. In addition, pseudo-label was performed to optimize the decision boundary. The experimental results show that our method does improve the classification accuracy of B-lymphoblast cells and achieves better results than the mainstream convolutional neural network.

References

1. Krizhevsky, A., Hinton, G.: Learning multiple layers of features from tiny images. Technical report, Citeseer (2009)
2. Krizhevsky, A., Sutskever, I., Hinton, G.E.: ImageNet classification with deep convolutional neural networks. In: Advances in Neural Information Processing Systems, pp. 1097–1105 (2012)
3. Fu, H., Xu, Y., Wong, D.W.K., Liu, J.: Retinal vessel segmentation via deep learning network and fully-connected conditional random fields. In: 2016 IEEE 13th International Symposium on Biomedical Imaging (ISBI), pp. 698–701 (2016). https://doi.org/10.1109/ISBI.2016.7493362
4. Huang, X., Shan, J., Vaidya, V.: Lung nodule detection in CT using 3D convolutional neural networks. In: 2017 IEEE 14th International Symposium on Biomedical Imaging (ISBI 2017), pp. 379–383 (2017). https://doi.org/10.1109/ISBI.2017.7950542
5. Habibzadeh, M., Jannesari, M., Rezaei, Z., Baharvand, H., Totonchi, M.: Automatic white blood cell classification using pre-trained deep learning models: ResNet and inception. In: Tenth International Conference on Machine Vision (ICMV 2017), vol. 10696, p. 1069612. International Society for Optics and Photonics (2018)
6. Yosinski, J., Clune, J., Nguyen, A., Fuchs, T., Lipson, H.: Understanding neural networks through deep visualization (2015). arXiv:1506.06579
7. Russakovsky, O., Deng, J., Su, H., Krause, J., Satheesh, S., Ma, S., Huang, Z., Karpathy, A., Khosla, A., Bernstein, M., et al.: Imagenet large scale visual recognition challenge. Int. J. Comput. Vis. **115**(3), 211–252 (2015)
8. Lee, D.H.: Pseudo-label: the simple and efficient semi-supervised learning method for deep neural networks. In: Workshop on Challenges in Representation Learning, ICML, vol. 3, p. 2 (2013)
9. Young, I.T.: The classification of white blood cells. IEEE Trans. Biomed. Eng. **4**, 291–298 (1972)
10. Faraki, M., Harandi, M.T., Wiliem, A., Lovell, B.C.: Fisher tensors for classifying human epithelial cells. Pattern Recognit. **47**(7), 2348–2359 (2014)
11. Kong, X., Li, K., Cao, J., Yang, Q., Wenyin, L.: HEp-2 cell pattern classification with discriminative dictionary learning. Pattern Recognit. **47**(7), 2379–2388 (2014)
12. LeCun, Y., Bottou, L., Bengio, Y., Haffner, P., et al.: Gradient-based learning applied to document recognition. Proc. IEEE **86**(11), 2278–2324 (1998)
13. Bayramoglu, N., Kannala, J., Heikkilä, J.: Human epithelial type 2 cell classification with convolutional neural networks. In: 2015 IEEE 15th International Conference on Bioinformatics and Bioengineering (BIBE), pp. 1–6. IEEE (2015)
14. Lei, H., Han, T., Zhou, F., Yu, Z., Qin, J., Elazab, A., Lei, B.: A deeply supervised residual network for HEp-2 cell classification via cross-modal transfer learning. Pattern Recognit. **79**, 290–302 (2018)
15. Xue, Y., Ray, N.: Output encoding by compressed sensing for cell detection with deep convnet. In: Workshops at the Thirty-Second AAAI Conference on Artificial Intelligence (2018)
16. Duggal, R., Gupta, A., Gupta, R., Mallick, P.: SD-layer: stain deconvolutional layer for CNNs in medical microscopic imaging. In: International Conference on Medical Image Computing and Computer-Assisted Intervention, pp. 435–443. Springer (2017)
17. He, K., Zhang, X., Ren, S., Sun, J.: Deep residual learning for image recognition. In: Proceedings of the IEEE Conference on Computer Vision and Pattern Recognition, pp. 770–778 (2016)
18. Simonyan, K., Zisserman, A.: Very deep convolutional networks for large-scale image recognition (2014). arXiv:1409.1556
19. Zhang, H., Xue, J., Dana, K.: Deep ten: texture encoding network. In: Proceedings of the IEEE Conference on Computer Vision and Pattern Recognition, pp. 708–717 (2017)
20. Huang, G., Liu, Z., Van Der Maaten, L., Weinberger, K.Q.: Densely connected convolutional networks. In: Proceedings of the IEEE Conference on Computer Vision and Pattern Recognition, pp. 4700–4708 (2017)

21. Chen, Y., Li, J., Xiao, H., Jin, X., Yan, S., Feng, J.: Dual path networks. In: Advances in Neural Information Processing Systems, pp. 4467–4475 (2017)
22. Hu, J., Shen, L., Sun, G.: Squeeze-and-excitation networks. In: Proceedings of the IEEE Conference on Computer Vision and Pattern Recognition, pp. 7132–7141 (2018)
23. Szegedy, C., Ioffe, S., Vanhoucke, V., Alemi, A.A.: Inception-v4, inception-ResNet and the impact of residual connections on learning. In: Thirty-First AAAI Conference on Artificial Intelligence (2017)
24. Gupta, R., Mallick, P., Duggal, R., Gupta, A., Sharma, O.: Stain color normalization and segmentation of plasma cells in microscopic images as a prelude to development of computer assisted automated disease diagnostic tool in multiple myeloma. Clin. Lymphoma Myeloma Leukemia **17**(1), e99 (2017)
25. Duggal, R., Gupta, A., Gupta, R., Wadhwa, M., Ahuja, C.: Overlapping cell nuclei segmentation in microscopic images using deep belief networks. In: Proceedings of the Tenth Indian Conference on Computer Vision, Graphics and Image Processing, p. 82. ACM (2016)

Multi-streams and Multi-features for Cell Classification

Xinpeng Xie, Yuexiang Li, Menglu Zhang, Yong Wu and Linlin Shen

Abstract With the development of deep learning technique, cell classification has gained increasing interests from the community. Identifying malignant cells in B-ALL white blood cancer microscopic images is challenging, since the normal and malignant cells have similar appearances. Traditional cell identification approach requires experienced pathologists to carefully read the cell images, which is laborious and suffers from inter-observer variations. Hence, the computer aid diagnosis systems for blood disorders, for example, leukemia, are worthwhile to develop. In this paper, we design a multi-stream model to classify the immature leukemic blasts and normal cells. We evaluated the proposed model on the C-NMC 2019 challenge dataset. The experimental results show that a promising result is achieved by our model.

Keywords Leukemia cell identification · Deep learning network · Feature fusion

---

X. Xie · M. Zhang · Y. Wu · L. Shen (✉)
Computer Vision Institute, Shenzhen University, Shenzhen, Guangdong, China
e-mail: llshen@szu.edu.cn

X. Xie
e-mail: xiexinpeng2017@email.szu.edu.cn

M. Zhang
e-mail: 1810272064@email.szu.edu.cn

Y. Wu
e-mail: 2015130225@email.szu.edu.cn

Y. Li
Youtu Lab, Tencent, Shenzhen, China
e-mail: vicyxli@tencent.com

A. Gupta and R. Gupta (eds.), *ISBI 2019 C-NMC Challenge: Classification in Cancer Cell Imaging*, Lecture Notes in Bioengineering,
https://doi.org/10.1007/978-981-15-0798-4_10

1 Introduction

The B-acute lymphoblastic leukemia (B-ALL) leads to a number of possible symptoms and approximately 25% of the pediatric cancers [1]. Owing to the rapid growth, leukemia cells can divide and spread to replace the healthy cells that produce functional lymphocytes. Early diagnosis makes the patients achieve better treatment and thereby increases the overall survival rate. However, it is a challenging task for pathologists to classify the malignant cells from normal cells in B-ALL white blood cancer microscopic images, due to their similar appearances. The inter-observer variation may influence the leukemia diagnosis as well.

In order to achieve accurate identification of malignant cells, increasing number of works tried to apply deep learning technique to this area [2]. In the past several years, deep convolutional network achieves the state-of-the-art performances for the cell classification. Zhang et al. [3] extracted features from the raw cell data by a deep convolutional network for classification. Duggal et al. [4] proposed stain deconvolutional layer (SD layer) for cell classification in medical microscopic imaging. They transferred the original RGB image into the optical density (OD) space and combined the CNN architecture with an SD layer to learn the optimal stain basis vectors of cell of interest. Mourya et al. [5] introduced a multi-stage deep learning network to combine the discrete cosine transform (DCT) domain features with the optical density (OD) space features. The experimental result showed that the proposed framework is an effective "second-opinion" to help pathologists identify malignant cells.

In this paper, we design a multi-stream model to extract features for immature leukemic blasts and normal cells classification. The main contributions of this work are listed in the following:

(1) We try different pre-processing approaches on the training set, for example, transferring the RGB image into HSV space, and fuse the inside and outside features for better classification.
(2) We develop an effective framework based on Inception ResNetV2 for the leukemic cells classification, which achieves competitive results on ISBI 2019 competition: classification of normal versus malignant cells in B-ALL white blood cancer microscopic images.

2 Dataset Description

2.1 Dataset

The C-NMC 2019 challenge dataset [6] is adopted in this study. The dataset contains 10,661 pieces of microscopic images extracted from the bone marrow aspirate slides of normal and B-ALL subjects. All the images were normalized using [7, 8] for stain variation. Cells have been segmented using [9, 10] from the microscopic images

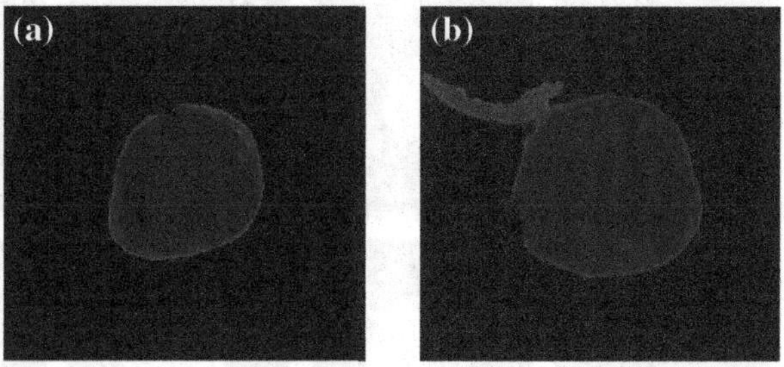

Fig. 1 Example images from C-NMC dataset. **a** and **b** are the nucleus of normal/malignant cell, respectively

collected from the patients and embedded in a 450 × 450 black-colored patch to avoid texture alteration. In total, the dataset constitutes 7272 cancer cells from 47 subjects and 3389 normal cells from 29 subjects. Example images from the dataset are shown in Fig. 1. In addition, another 1867 images collected from 30 subjects are adopted as test set, which consists of 1219 cancer cells from 15 cancer subjects and 648 normal cells from 15 normal subjects.

2.2 *Pre-processing*

We separate the dataset into training and validation sets according to the ratio of 70:30 at subject level instead of image level. All cells belonging to the same subject are placed under the same fold to ensure that the images of validation sets are untouched.

Since the dataset is small and imbalanced, we applied data augmentation approaches, such as random rotation, horizontal and vertical flip, during the training phase, which results in an augmented balanced dataset. We also tried various augmentations, such as color adjustment, Gaussian blur, random crop and elastic transform. The last two operations provide obvious improvement in our experiments.

In addition, we also try to transfer the RGB image to HSV space for clear observation of cell features. Some examples are shown in Fig. 2. HSV images provide us a new view to learn cell features; for example, it is more likely to observe the texture information of cells in S channel.

3 Network Architecture

The flowchart of our classification framework is shown in Fig. 3. This is a three-stream network. The features extracted by each basic network are concatenated together and then fed into multi-layer perception (MLP) to get the final classification result. The resolution of C-NMC 2019 challenge dataset is 450 × 450. Since the interest of cell is easy to segment, we conduct three different ways to prepare the training set: (i) resize the image into 299 × 299 directly (referred to "outside image"); (ii) crop

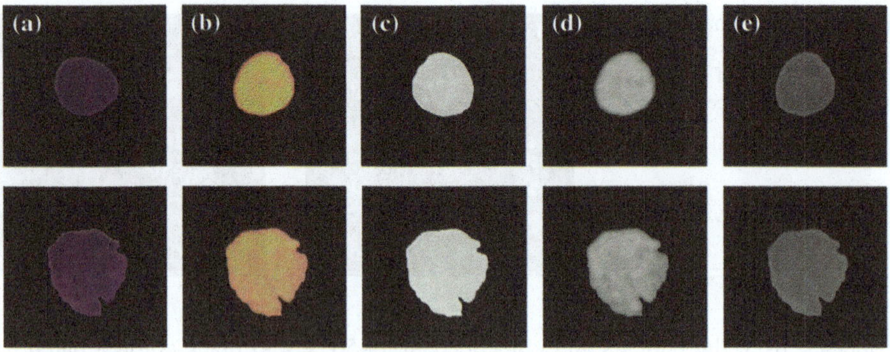

Fig. 2 Examples of transferred HSV images. **a–e** represent the original RGB image, HSV image, H channel, S channel, V channel image, respectively

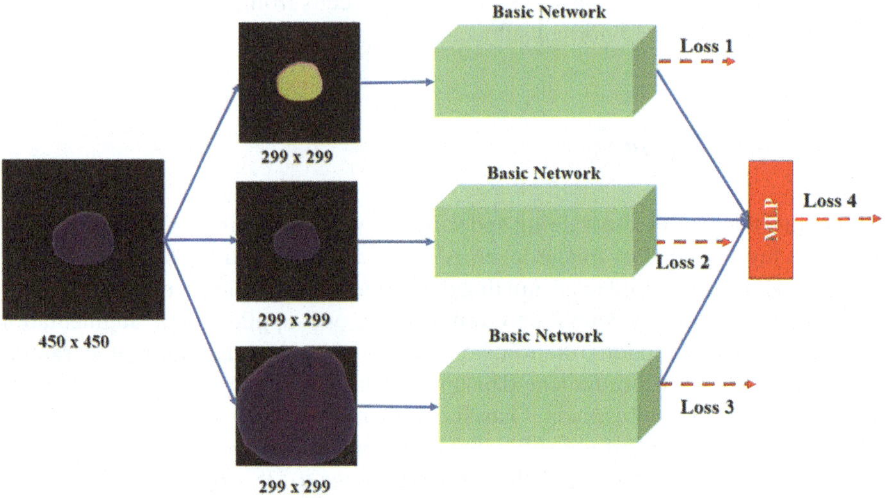

Fig. 3 The framework of our classification model

the interest of cell and then resize it to 299 × 299 (referred to "interest image") and (iii) transfer the RGB image to HSV space and then resize it to 299 × 299 (referred to "HSV image"). In our experiment, we find that the "interest image" provides bigger contribution for learning the inside texture belonged to malignant cell area/normal cell, while the "outside image" is prone to represent the outside information like shape or boundary of cell. The "HSV image" is introduced to enhance the ability of network to extract enough texture information for classification.

Inception ResNetV2. Once the training sets are prepared, we feed them into different streams network for feature extraction. The residual connections [11] are adopted in our framework. The Inception [12] architecture has achieved very good performance at relatively low computational cost. In our study, we adopt the Inception ResNetV2 [13] as our basic network. Finally, we ensemble multiple models to further improve the performance of classification.

4 Experiments

4.1 Implementation

The proposed framework is implemented using Keras toolbox. The network is trained with a mini-batch size of 64 on four GPUs (GeForce GTX TITAN X, 12 GB RAM). Size of input is 299 × 299. The initial learning rate is set to 0.0001. The network was optimized using "Adam" [14] and supervised with cross-entropy loss.

4.2 Evaluation Criterion

The F1 score of all the test images is adopted as the criterion for performance evaluation. It can be expressed in terms of statistical measures as:

$$F_1 = 2 \cdot \frac{\text{precision} \cdot \text{recall}}{\text{precision} + \text{recall}}$$

4.3 Feature Visualization

To have a better understanding of which part of the cell exactly makes contribution for cell type classification, we visualize the features extracted by the last convolutional layer of Inception ResNetV2 on the C-NMC 2019 challenge dataset. As depicted in Fig. 4, the feature extracted from the "interest image" is more likely to represent the texture information of the whole cell, while the feature of the "outside image" indicates the shape or boundary information of cell. The feature of the "HSV image" makes a supplement to the information for classification.

4.4 Experimental Results

The C-NMC 2019 challenge dataset is imbalanced with the ratio of malignant/normal cells of about 2:1, which may cause the fluctuated performance on classifying cells.

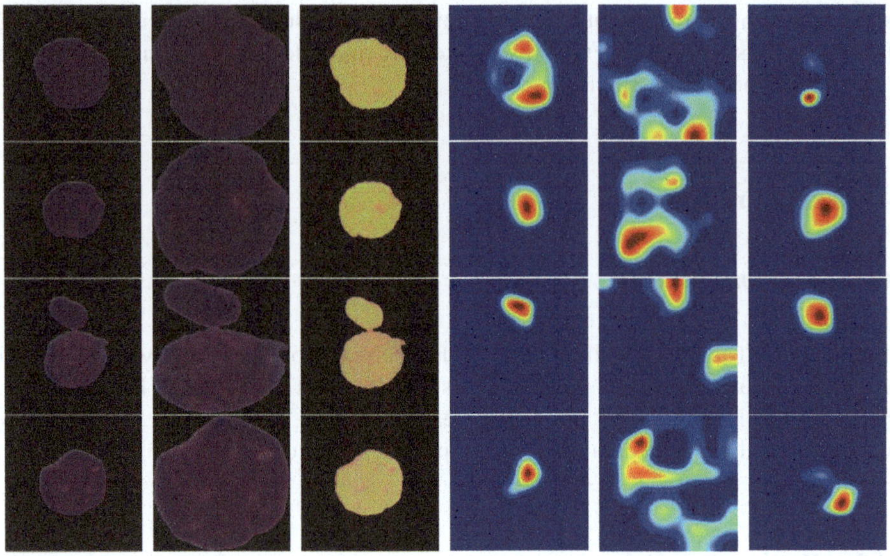

Fig. 4 Visualization of the feature heatmaps extracted from the Inception ResNetV2. The first three columns are the "outside image", "interest image", "HSV image" and the last three columns are the features extracted from them, respectively

We adopt data augmentations, such as rotation, flip and randomly crop the data, to make the number of normal cells basically equal to the number of malignant cells. This results in a more stable training and an increase of about 2% in accuracy on classifying cells, that is, improve the F1 score from 82.31 to 84.75% on test set. We test the performance of the Inception ResNetV2 trained with different data preparation ways. The F1 scores on validation and testing sets are summarized in Table 1. The "outside image" and the "interest image" stand for the image resized and cropped from the original image, respectively. The "HSV image" refers to the image transferred from the RGB image. It can be observed from Table 1 that the model trained with different datasets achieves basically the same performance on cell classification. While fusing the feature extracted from different datasets together, the F1 score on validation and testing sets has significantly improved from 89.94 to 90.32% and from 85.91 to 88.54%, respectively. This demonstrates that feature fusion leads to a network with better generalization.

Table 1 F1 scores of Inception ResNetV2 with different data preparation ways (%)

Training data	Validation set	Testing set
Outside image	87.88	83.98
Interest image	**89.94**	**85.91**
HSV image	89.04	84.73
Fusion	**90.32**	**88.54**

Table 2 F1 scores for Top-6 (%)

Model	F1 score (%)
Top 1	88.91
Top 2	88.69
Top 3	88.12
Top 4	87.64
Top 5	84.26
Top 6 (Ours)	**83.35**

C-NMC 2019 Challenge Result. We achieve a competitive F1 score with 83.35% on the ISBI2019 competition test set, while the highest score is 88.91%. Table 2 listed the Top-6 results on the leaderboard.

5 Conclusion

In this work, we present a multi-stream and multi-feature architecture for the classification of normal and malignant cells in B-ALL white blood cancer microscopic images. We adopt the Inception ResNetV2 as our basic network and employ a hybrid architecture that utilizes the knowledge of three basic networks. Augmentations and class balance improve the classification accuracy. We fuse the features of different datasets together to provide the network stronger generalization performance. The proposed framework is evaluated on publicly available C-NMC 2019 challenge dataset and achieves a promising result on cell classification task.

References

1. Bhojwani, D., Yang, J.J., Pui, C.-H.: Biology of childhood acute lymphoblastic leukemia. Pediatr. Clin. **62**(1), 47–60 (2015)
2. Roth, H.R., Lee, C.T., Shin, H.C., Seff, A., Kim, L., Yao, J., Lu, L., Summers, R.M.: Anatomy-specific classification of medical images using deep convolutional nets. In: IEEE International Symposium on Biomedical Imaging, pp. 101–104 (2015)
3. Zhang, L., Lu, L., Nogues, I., et al.: DeepPap: deep convolutional networks for cervical cell classification. IEEE J. Biomed. Health Inf. **21**(6), 1633–1643 (2017)
4. Duggal, R., Gupta, A., Gupta, R., et al.: SD-layer: stain deconvolutional layer for CNNs in medical microscopic imaging. In: International Conference on Medical Image Computing and Computer-Assisted Intervention. Springer, Cham (2017)
5. Mourya, S., Kant, S., Kumar, P., Gupta, A., et al.: LeukoNet: DCT-based CNN architecture for the classification of normal versus Leukemic blasts in B-ALL Cancer (2018). arXiv:1810.07961
6. Classification of Normal vs Malignant Cells in B-ALL White Blood Cancer Microscopic Images: ISBI 2019. https://competitions.codalab.org/competitions/20429

7. Gupta, A., Duggal, R., Gupta, R., Kumar, L., Thakkar, N., Satpathy, D.: GCTI-SN: Geometry-Inspired Chemical and Tissue Invariant Stain Normalization of Microscopic Medical Images. Under review
8. Gupta, R., Mallick, P., Duggal, R., Gupta, A., Sharma, O.: Stain color normalization and segmentation of plasma cells in microscopic images as a prelude to development of computer assisted automated disease diagnostic tool in multiple Myeloma. In: 16th International Myeloma Workshop, India, March (2017)
9. Duggal, R., Gupta, A., Gupta, R., Wadhwa, M., Ahuja, C.: Overlapping cell nuclei segmentation in microscopic images using deep belief networks. In: Indian Conference on Computer Vision, Graphics and Image Processing, India, December (2016)
10. Duggal, R., Gupta, A., Gupta, R.: Segmentation of overlapping/touching white blood cell nuclei using artificial neural networks. CME Series on HematoOncopathology, All India Institute of Medical Sciences, New Delhi, India, July (2016)
11. He, K., Zhang, X., Ren, S., et al.: Deep residual learning for image recognition. In: Proceedings of the IEEE Conference on Computer Vision and Pattern Recognition (2016)
12. Szegedy, C., Vanhoucke, V., Ioffe, S., et al.: Rethinking the inception architecture for computer vision. In: Proceedings of the IEEE Conference on Computer Vision and Pattern Recognition (2016)
13. Szegedy, C., Ioffe, S., Vanhoucke, V., et al.: Inception-v4, Inception-ResNet and the impact of residual connections on learning. In: Thirty-First AAAI Conference on Artificial Intelligence (2017)
14. Kingma, D.P., Ba, J.: Adam: A method for stochastic optimization (2014). arXiv:1412.6980

Classification of Normal Versus Malignant Cells in B-ALL Microscopic Images Based on a Tiled Convolution Neural Network Approach

Pouyan Mohajerani and Vasilis Ntziachristos

Abstract In this paper we present a method based on the existing convolution neural network architecture of AlexNet for the purpose of classifying microscopic images of B-ALL white blood cancer cells. This classification problem is especially challenging due to lack of conspicuous morphological differences between normal and malignant cell nuclei. Therefore, we designed a machine learning pipeline that focused on the texture of the staining images. Briefly, our approach divides the cell image into several overlapping tiles and trains a modified version of AlexNet on the tiles. Only those tiles are retained which are fully contained within the cell image. Several such networks were trained in an ensemble fashion using different training–validation data splits. For a given test image, the tiles are generated and ran through all the trained networks. The outputs of all networks along with the nucleus area are then fed into a simple decision tree, which generates the final prediction. The proposed method was developed in the context of the ISBI 2019 C-NMC challenge. The final testing results demonstrated a classification-weighted F1 score of 0.8307 using 2586 test images. The results demonstrate the possibility of making relatively accurate predictions using only local texture features.

Keywords Convolution neural network · Machine learning · Deep learning · Cell classification · Acute lymphoblastic leukemia

1 Introduction

Deep learning methods, particularly based on convolutional neural network (CNN) architectures, are being widely applied in pathology and toward automated evaluation of histology images and image cytometry [1–6]. Applications of deep learning methods on histology images or the genetic profile of the patient include cell classification [2–4] and clinical survival outcome prediction [5, 6].

P. Mohajerani (✉) · V. Ntziachristos
Chair of Biological Imaging, Technische Universität München, Munich, Germany
e-mail: pouyan.mohajerani@gmail.com

Institute of Biological and Medical Imaging, Helmholtz Zentrum München, Neuherberg, Germany

A. Gupta and R. Gupta (eds.), *ISBI 2019 C-NMC Challenge: Classification in Cancer Cell Imaging*, Lecture Notes in Bioengineering,
https://doi.org/10.1007/978-981-15-0798-4_11

Acute lymphoblastic leukemia (ALL) is a type of blood cell cancer and is one the most common forms of leukemia, which is associated with the development of immature lymphocytes, mostly affecting children between 2 and 5 years of age [7]. Automatic detection of malignant immature white blood cells using histology images and their differentiation from the benign cells is a challenging problem, which has been previously investigated using conventional machine learning approaches based on feature engineering [8, 9]. Deep learning methods have been further recently proposed for this task [10, 11]. In particular, a method is presented in [10] to preprocess the color space using a layer placed at the beginning of the CNN, which is expected to improve the classification accuracy, as the existing pretrained CNN architectures are often developed for the RGB color space of natural images.

In this paper we present an ensemble approach based on a modified version of AlexNet [12] which relies mainly on the image texture for classification purposes. Briefly, the cell images are portioned into overlapping tiles, which are then used for training the networks. In the execution phase, several networks are run on the extracted tiles (of a given test image) and their mirrored versions (as a form of execution-phase augmentation) and the results are pooled and fed into a small decision tree, which also uses the cell area as an input to generate the final prediction. The current work was developed in the context of the ISBI 2019 C-NMC challenge. The training and evaluation were performed using, respectively, 10,661 and 2586 images of segmented cell nuclei, labeled and provided by the Signal Processing and Biomedical Imaging Lab (SBILab), at Indian Institute of Technology Delhi [10, 13–16], Delhi, India. The results of predictions performed over the 2586 test images manifested a weighted F1 score of 0.8307.

2 The Proposed Methodology

As a first step toward designing a machine learning solution for this classification problem, we examined transfer learning using pretrained networks on whole images. This approach did not lend satisfactory results. Instead, we obtained better results by training networks on tiles, defined by a small square portion of the original images. In this way we are limiting the classification to texture only.

2.1 Training–Validation Splitting

Throughout this work the separation of data into training and validation subsets was performed at the subject level. The entire training dataset consisted of 10,661 images from a total of 47 cancerous subject (with label `all`) and 26 healthy subjects (with label `hem`). To create a training–validation set, 80% of the subjects are selected from each of the classes at random and their data are pooled into the training set. The rest are assigned to the validation set. We created different training–validation splits and trained several networks. In this way we can achieve a form of cross-validation. The networks are then pooled together in an ensemble fashion. The evaluation set consists of the test images released by the challenge organizers (with true labels unbeknownst to us).

2.2 *The Machine Learning Pipeline*

The developed machine learning pipeline is shown in Fig. 1. Specifically, first the images were morphologically opened [17] using a structural element of size 25 to remove residual components from the remaining previous segmentation module. Next, a dataset of image tiles was generated as follows. Each image was divided into several (on average around 20) overlapping tiles of size $60 \times 60 \times 3$. Only tiles which were fully contained in the original image (i.e. contained no black parts) were retained. These steps are depicted graphically in Fig. 2. This operation resulted in a dataset of around 200,000 labeled 60×60 RBG images. The tiles had an overlap of 30 for the positive images and an overlap of 16 for the negative images. This label-based selection of the overlap was done to compensate for the class imbalance existing in the training dataset (68% positive, 32% negative). In this way the tiled dataset has balanced classes. The tiles were further downsampled by a factor of 2 to sizes 30×30 for memory management purposes. This downsampling did not result in any noticeable visual degradation.

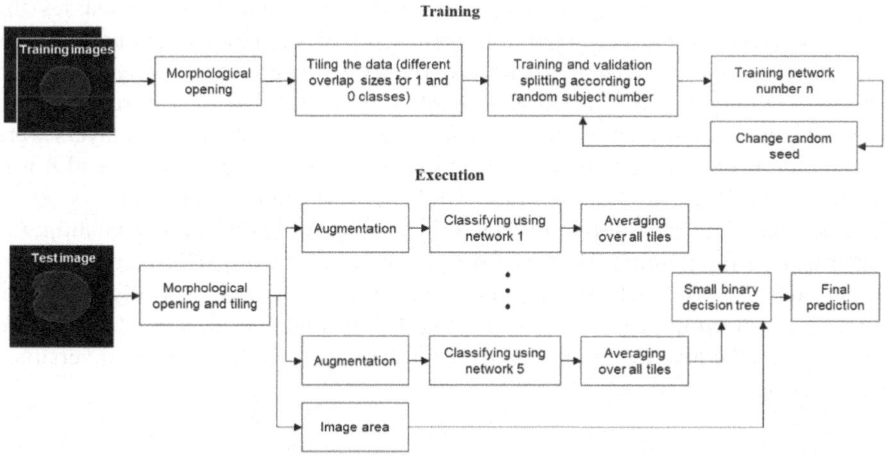

Fig. 1 The machine learning pipeline: upper row is the training pipeline and low row shows the execution phase. During the training, five CNN networks are trained in an ensemble fashion using the same set of hyperparameters, but with different subsets of the entire training set. During the execution, the image is first morphologically opened and then tiled. The tiles are fed to all five networks and the outputs are fed to a decision tree, which generates the final prediction

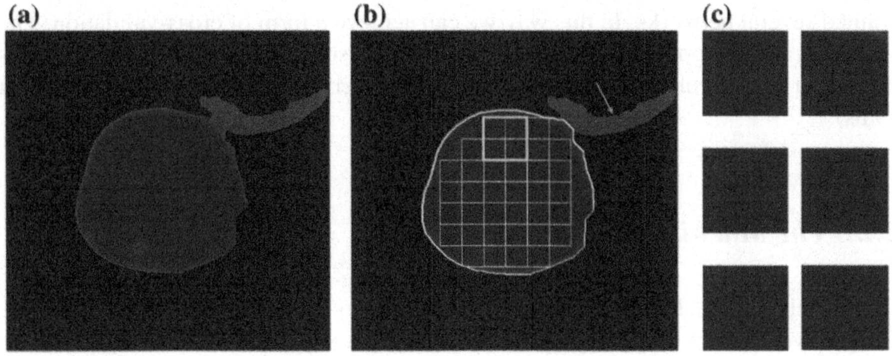

Fig. 2 The preprocessing steps of the machine learning pipeline. **a** Sample input image. **b** The orange arrow points to the image component which is likely due to imperfect segmentation. This component is removed via morphological opening, leaving the main component, encompassed by the white boundary. The yellow squares show 24 tiles of size 60 × 60 in this image, with overlaps equal to half an edge length. For clarity, one square is highlighted with cyan color. **c** Six tiles extracted from this image. Each tile has a size of 30 × 30, which results from further downsampling by a factor of ×2. This downsampling resulted in no degradation

Subsequently, a CNN network based on the AlexNet [12] was trained on this new dataset. The input images were resized from 30 × 30 × 3 to 227 × 227 × 3 (as AlexNet has an input size of 227 × 227 × 3). The last two fully connected (FC) layers of AlexNet, that is, fc6 and fc7 layers, each with 4096 output nodes, were changed to FC layers with 8 and 5 input nodes. This modification in the architecture is justified, as we have only two classes and AlexNet was trained for 1000 classes (the last FC layer, i.e. fc8, was changed from 1000 nodes to two nodes, as our problem has only two classes). Five such networks were trained with different training–validation subsets. Training was performed with ADAM optimizer. The data were reshuffled after each epoch. Different combinations of the first few convolutional layers were frozen (and set to their original values in the AlexNet). However, at the end it was decided that end-to-end training of the whole network lends better result.

Other than the generation of overlapping tiles, no further data augmentation was performed during training. However, data augmentation was performed in the execution phase, where each tile was mirrored horizontally and vertically. The final output for a given image and a given network was a number between 0 and 1 and calculated as the average prediction over all the tiles (and their mirrored versions) for that image.

2.3 *Pooling the Predictions of the Networks*

The results of the five networks were polled using a simple manually designed binary decision tree, which also had the (original, untiled) image area as the input. The image area slightly improved the results as negative images are generally smaller than positive images. Let p_i, $i = 1, \ldots, 5$ be a real number between 0 and 1, denoting the prediction of the network number i on a given test image (averaged over all the tiles and their vertically and horizontally mirrored versions). Therefore, $p_i = 0.9$ means the network i predicted a positive label for 90% of the tiles extracted from a given image (also counting the mirrored versions). Also, let a denote the area of the morphologically opened image in pixels. The final prediction is given as

$$p = \underbrace{((\max(p_1, p_2, p_3) > th_1 \wedge a > A_1) \vee a > A_2)}_{q_1} \wedge \underbrace{\max(p_4, p_5) > th_2}_{q_2}, \quad (1)$$

where $\wedge$ and $\vee$ denote logical `AND` and `OR` operations, respectively. Equation (1) is indeed a small decision tree, built on the top of the five networks. This tree is heuristically designed using the training data released in the first round of the competition. The same exact tree was used for both of the round 2 and round 3 predictions, resulting in 0.84 and 0.83, weighted F1 scores, respectively. These results rule out overfitting in this decision tree.

Equation (1) can be interpreted and justified as follows. The term q_1 is `true` if the image area is very large (A_2 set to 49,000, as marked on the histogram of Fig. 3) OR if any of the first three networks predicted with a very high certainty ($th_1 = 0.91$) that the cell is malignant. The threshold th_2 in the term q_2 is set to the small value of 0.1. Therefore, q_2 is `true` if at least the other two networks (numbers 4 and 5) have seen some evidence of malignancy. Also, the term $a > A_1$ in q_1 ascertains that any image with total size of $A_1 = 22{,}000$ or less is normal. The thresholds A_1 and A_2 were set using the histograms shown in Fig. 3. The thresholds th_1 and th_2 were set manually using the overall accuracy over the entire training set.

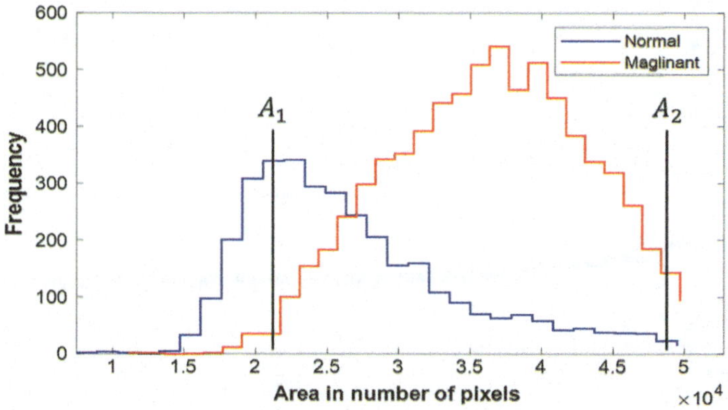

Fig. 3 Red and blue curves denote the image area histograms of normal and malignant cells, respectively. Although the normal and malignant cells showed no particular morphological features, image area did show some discriminative power, as the malignant cells are generally larger. The two thresholds A_1 and A_2 are used later to design a decision tree which sits atop an ensemble of CNNs ($A_1 = 22{,}000$, $A_2 = 49{,}000$)

2.4 *Evaluation Criterion*

The prediction performance was evaluated using the weighted F1 score which yields a harmonic mean of the precision and recall, weighted for the class imbalance (a mathematical definition of the weighted F1 score, as used by scikit-learn is presented in Ref. [18]). The processing was performed using neural networks toolbox of MATLAB, version 2018b (The MathWorks Inc., USA), on a PC equipped with Nvidia's GTX 1080 Ti graphic card.

3 Results

As noted above, five networks were trained using different training–validation splits (performed on the subject level). Figure 4 presents the learning curves for one of the networks, with the upper graph showing the accuracy and the lower graph depicting the loss. The training curves are showing with blue and orange colors, while the validation curves are marked with black circles.

The networks had varying final accuracies (as shown in the example presented in Fig. 4, the final validation accuracy was around 0.76). Nevertheless, the final predictions had a weighted F1 score of 0.83. This improvement in classification

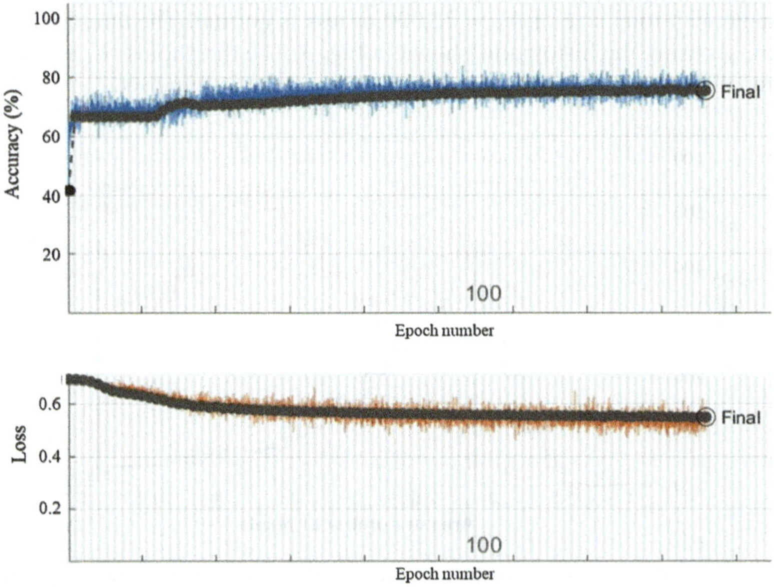

Fig. 4 Learning curves of one of the trained networks. The red and blue curves corresponding to training set and the dotted curves to validation set. Upper and lower panels show accuracy and loss, respectively. Alternating vertical gray and white bars denote epochs

accuracy is due to ensemble nature of the entire pipeline, where the predictions of the networks are combined in the decision tree, as explained in Sect. 2.3.

The decision tree shown in Eq. (1) was observed to consistently yield an accuracy of at least 0.83 (as observed by performing prediction on the test data of both second and third rounds of the Challenge). Nevertheless, it should be noted that only the first term of Eq. (1), that is $\max(p_1, p_2, p_3) > th_1$, was observed to have a significant contribution to the overall prediction accuracy. The rest of the terms did improve the performance, however, in a marginal fashion.

4 Discussion and Conclusion

The major challenge in this work, as is generally expected, was that of overfitting. There were 10,661 labeled images available, belonging to a total of 76 subjects. The images for each given subject are expected to correlate. This renders the effective size of the dataset smaller than the total number of labeled samples. To reduce overfitting, training and validation data were chosen on the subject level, that is from different subjects (or patients), according to a preset proportion of 80–20% for each class.

The specific training–validation split chosen was observed to affect the prediction accuracy. In other words, we observed that it is possible to create a "hard" split, for which the training fails (i.e. the validation accuracy is low). One such split is presented in Fig. 5. As seen in this figure, the network has quickly overfitted, discernable by the close-to-random accuracy on the validation set (the dotted black curve). To improve the accuracy of our final model, we focused on such hard splits to improve and chose the network architecture and hyperparameters.

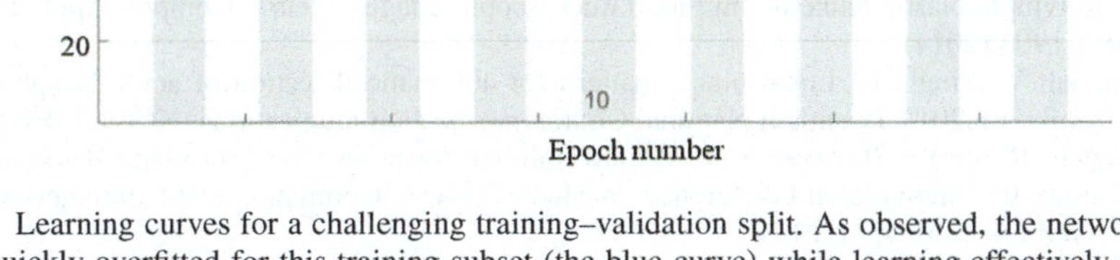

Fig. 5 Learning curves for a challenging training–validation split. As observed, the network has been quickly overfitted for this training subset (the blue curve) while learning effectively almost nothing at all (as seen in the validation accuracy of around 50% by the dotted black curve). We focused on such "hard" training–validation splits, to improve the hyperparameters. Alternating vertical gray and white bars denote epochs

One important point for further improvement is that we resized our 30 × 30 × 3 image tiles to match the input size of AlexNet (227 × 227 × 3). This is not an efficient approach, as we do not use the whole input scope of AlexNet. Theoretically, it should be possible to obtain the same results (or even improved performance) by using smaller CNNs which mimic AlexNet for smaller images. This way, we can also achieve very fast execution time due to the small number of parameters (and needed operations) in the small networks.

Overall, we presented a relatively straightforward approach for classification of ALL versus normal blood cells. Our method used a modified version of the existing AlexNet architecture and performed the predictions of the square-shaped subsections of the RGB images. Nevertheless, we achieved a fairly good prediction accuracy of 0.83 for the test set. These results show that it is possible to achieve classification by focusing only on the local texture features. Our method can be combined with other methods in an ensemble learning fashion to improve the overall accuracy of this cell classification task. Furthermore, applying preprocessing layers to transform the color space, as proposed in [10], might further improve the accuracy of our method.

References

1. Gupta, A., et al.: Deep learning in image cytometry: a review. Cytom. Part A (2018)
2. Cruz-Roa, A.A., et al.: A Deep Learning Architecture for Image Representation, Visual Interpretability and Automated Basal-Cell Carcinoma Cancer Detection. Springer, Berlin (2013)
3. Bayramoglu, N., Kannala, J., Heikkilä, J.: Deep learning for magnification independent breast cancer histopathology image classification. In: 2016 23rd International Conference on Pattern Recognition (ICPR). IEEE (2016)
4. Cireşan, D.C., et al.: Mitosis detection in breast cancer histology images with deep neural networks. In: International Conference on Medical Image Computing and Computer-assisted Intervention. Springer (2013)
5. Mobadersany, P., et al.: Predicting cancer outcomes from histology and genomics using convolutional networks. Proc. Natl. Acad. Sci. **115**(13), E2970–E2979 (2018)
6. Yousefi, S., et al.: Predicting clinical outcomes from large scale cancer genomic profiles with deep survival models. Sci. Rep. **7**(1), 11707 (2017)
7. Inaba, H., Greaves, M., Mullighan, C.G.: Acute lymphoblastic leukaemia. The Lancet **381**(9881), 1943–1955 (2013)
8. Mohapatra, S., Patra, D., Satpathy, S.: An ensemble classifier system for early diagnosis of acute lymphoblastic leukemia in blood microscopic images. Neural Comput. Appl. **24**(7–8), 1887–1904 (2014)
9. Singhal, V., Singh, P.: Local binary pattern for automatic detection of acute lymphoblastic leukemia. In: 2014 Twentieth National Conference on Communications (NCC). IEEE (2014)
10. Duggal, R., et al.: SD-layer: stain deconvolutional layer for CNNs in medical microscopic imaging. In: International Conference on Medical Image Computing and Computer-Assisted Intervention. Springer (2017)
11. Zhao, J., et al.: Automatic detection and classification of leukocytes using convolutional neural networks. Med. Biol. Eng. Comput. **55**(8), 1287–1301 (2017)
12. Krizhevsky, A., Sutskever, I., Hinton, G.E.: Imagenet classification with deep convolutional neural networks. In: Advances in Neural Information Processing Systems (2012)
13. Gupta, A., et al.: GCTI-SN: Geometry-Inspired Chemical and Tissue Invariant Stain Normalization of Microscopic Medical Images

14. Gupta, R., et al.: Stain color normalization and segmentation of plasma cells in microscopic images as a prelude to development of computer assisted automated disease diagnostic tool in multiple Myeloma. Clin. Lymphoma Myeloma Leuk. **17**(1), e99 (2017)
15. Duggal, R., et al.: Overlapping cell nuclei segmentation in microscopic images using deep belief networks. In: Proceedings of the Tenth Indian Conference on Computer Vision, Graphics and Image Processing. ACM (2016)
16. Duggal, R., Gupta, A., Gupta, R.: Segmentation of overlapping/touching white blood cell nuclei using artificial neural networks. In CME Series on Hemato-Oncopathology, All India Institute of Medical Sciences (AIIMS). New Delhi, India (2016)
17. Woods, G.A.: Digital Image Processing (2008)
18. https://spark.apache.org/docs/2.2.0/mllib-evaluation-metrics.html

Acute Lymphoblastic Leukemia Cells Image Analysis with Deep Bagging Ensemble Learning

Ying Liu and Feixiao Long

Abstract Acute lymphoblastic leukemia (ALL) is a blood cancer that leads to 111,000 death globally in 2015. Recently, diagnosing ALL often involves the microscopic image analysis with the help of deep learning (DL) techniques. However, as most medical related problems, deficiency training samples and minor visual difference between ALL and normal cells make the image analysis task quite challenging. Herein, an augmented image enhanced bagging ensemble learning with elaborately designed training subsets were proposed to tackle the above challenges. The weighted F_1-scores of the preliminary test set and final test are 0.84 and 0.88, respectively employing our ensemble model predictions and ranked within the top 10% in ISBI-2019 Classification of Normal versus Malignant White Blood Cancer Cells contest. Our results preliminarily demonstrate the efficacy of employing DL based techniques in ALL cells image analysis.

Keywords All cells classification · Deep learning · Enhanced bagging ensemble method

1 Introduction

Acute lymphoblastic leukemia (ALL) is a blood cell cancer caused by the development of immature lymphocytes. About 876,000 people suffer ALL globally in 2015 and lead to 111,000 death according to the data shown in [1]. The treatment of ALL

The pre-print is online: Y. Liu and F. Long, Acute lymphoblastic leukemia cells image analysis with deep bagging ensemble learning, bioRxiv, 2019, doi: https://doi.org/10.1101/580852.

Y. Liu
College of Statistics, University of International Business and Economics, Beijing 100029, China

F. Long (✉)
Hudongfeng Technology (Beijing) Co., Ltd., Beijing 100024, China
e-mail: lf832003@gmail.com

A. Gupta and R. Gupta (eds.), *ISBI 2019 C-NMC Challenge: Classification in Cancer Cell Imaging*, Lecture Notes in Bioengineering,
https://doi.org/10.1007/978-981-15-0798-4_12

normally includes chemotherapy which may last for several years. Typically, diagnosis of ALL is through blood tests and bone marrow biopsy, etc. Among several tests, microscopic image-based inspection is one of the promising and easy implemented methods, especially compared with expensive biochemical based inspections such as cell flow cytometry. The method through microscopic images to detect and classify various cells (not limited to ALL cells) can be viewed as a kind of well-defined and investigated computer vision (CV) problems. Recently, with the development of deep learning (DL) based techniques, researchers have investigated the potential use of applying DL methods in cell image classification problems. Compared with conventional handcraft features CV based solutions, DL based techniques have the advantages with automatically selecting representative image features of cells [13] and reduce the difficulty of solving ALL cells classification through a series of standard DL procedures.

For example, Shafique and Tehsin [10] employed upgraded Alex Net to differentiate ALL cells as well as their subtypes. Rehman et al. [8] also employed convolutional neural network (CNN) to classify ALL cells between normal cells. Besides, the authors compared the DL based methods to conventional machine learning (ML) approaches, such as k-nearest neighbors (k-NN), support vector machine (SVM), etc. Wang et al. [14] proposed a marker-based learning vector quantization neural network to detect and classify ALL cells.

However, although multiple researchers have shown the efficiency of applying DL based techniques in ALL cell image analysis, detecting ALL cells based on microscopic images would still be very challenging due to multiple reasons. First, in most medical-related object detection and classification problems, it requires professional medical knowledge or experiences to correctly label the objects. This often results in the deficiency training samples compared to nature image processing tasks. Second, to medical-related datasets, it is common to observe that the imbalance between the number of positive and negative or different categorical samples is due to the nature of disease or physiological situations. For example, the number of ALL cells is approximately twice the number of healthy cells (denoted as HEM) in the dataset (https://competitions.codalab.org/competitions/20429#learn_the_details-datadescription) employed in the experiment. From the aspect of machine learning, intuitively the imbalance issue will push the model to "learn" representative features from majority samples only and neglect minority ones without proper settings during training. Therefore, careful oversampling or undersampling of training sets, as well as other strategies, have to be performed in order to reduce the influences of imbalanced datasets. Last, as Fig. 1 shown, it is not easy to differentiate ALL and HEM cells images visually without professional experiences. In other words, the ALL cells discrimination problem suffers relative small inter-class similarity, which increases the difficulty of automatic detection.

In order to address the above issues, transfer learning [12] was employed to deal with relative deficiency training samples. Specifically, pretrained Inception ResNet V2 [11] using ImageNet (http://www.image-net.org) was employed as backbone net. Besides, a two-stage augmented image enhanced bagging ensemble training strategy [7] was employed to reduce the influences of imbalanced dataset. Two subsets (see

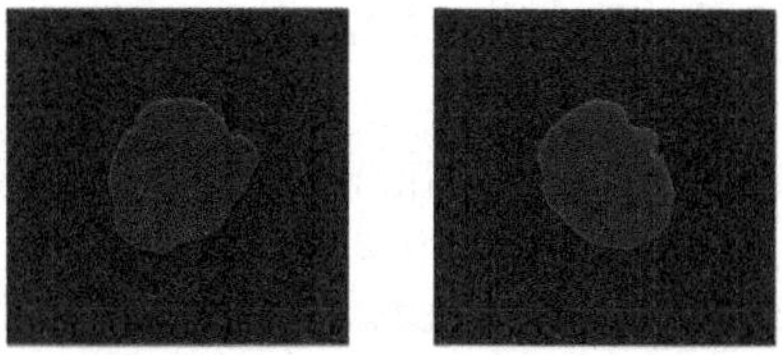

(a) ALL (b) Hem

Fig. 1 Close visual similarity between ALL and HEM cells

Sect. 2.3) were carefully designed for training backbone nets followed the idea shown in [7] in the first step training. Inspired by [16], two separately trained models were "combined" together and retrained with all training samples in order to further boost the overall prediction performance. Note that for simplicity, binary cross-entropy loss rather than the synergic loss was employed during the training of "combined" model.

The manuscript is arranged as follows: In the Methods section, our carefully designed training subsets will be described in detail. Moreover, the training settings and strategy will be discussed and introduced. In the Results section, the accuracy of the model will be illustrated. Finally, several issues of employing DL techniques in medical-related problems in the future will be discussed.

2 Methods

2.1 Details of Initial Dataset

As described in the contest (https://competitions.codalab.org/competitions/20429#learn_the_details) [2, 4], the initial dataset consists of 76 subjects, among which 47 subjects suffer ALL and the rest are healthy. Totally, there are 10,661 cells, in which 7,272 cells are classified as ALL and 3,389 cells are classified as HEM. Although there is only one cell in each training image, the image itself is not the convex hull of the cell and thus more black background than necessary is contained in the image. Herein segmentation of cells to get the convex hull through common image processing techniques was applied to the image (see Sect. 2.2) in order to get rid of the most black background. Staining and illumination error was still presented in the images although the artifacts were reduced by stain normalization techniques as shown in [3, 5, 6]. The initial dataset was then split into an original training set (see Sect. 2.3 for more details on generating final training set A and B) and validation set with proportion 7:3 as conventional settings in DL.

The preliminary test set consists of 30 subjects, in which 15 subjects are labeled as ALL and the rest are HEM. Similar cell segmentation and stain normalization techniques as described above were employed. In total, the preliminary test set consists of 1,867 cells, among which 1,219 cells were classified as ALL and 648 cells were HEM.

2.2 *Images Preprocessing*

As shown in [15], the authors employed a segmentation network first to segment the cell area from the image, making the classification network focus on representative and specific cell region [16] without being distracted by the background. Inspired by this idea, the cell images were first preprocessed through a series of image processing techniques to filter out most black background. Briefly, the RGB image was transferred to grayscale one and the region where the cells locate was binarized using the threshold estimated by Otsu's method followed by the erosion operation. The convex hull of the binarized region was then calculated and the RGB patch containing the cell in the middle was extracted accordingly. Finally, the image was resized to $299 \times 299 \times 3$ based on the input requirement of the employed backbone Inception ResNet [11] model.

2.3 *Training Dataset Generation*

Considering the number of ALL cells is approximately double of the number of HEM cells, we decided to adopt modified bagging ensemble training strategy [7] (briefly speaking two models employed, with each model learns different partial image features from majority classes but same features from minority classes intuitively) to deal with this imbalanced dataset and train the backbone models separately at the first stage training (see Sect. 2.5 for more details). The ALL cell samples were divided into two equal number subsets (named as "All-A" and "All-B", respectively, see Fig. 2). Moreover, randomly chosen one or a combination of several common image augmentation techniques, such as rotation, horizontal or vertical flip, Gaussian noise addition as well as contrast and color channel adjustment, etc., were applied to ALL cell subsets and HEM cell set for increasing the number of training samples and reducing over-fitting of the model. As shown in Fig. 2, the training set A consists of ALL samples from subset All-A and the augmentation images form subset All-B. In

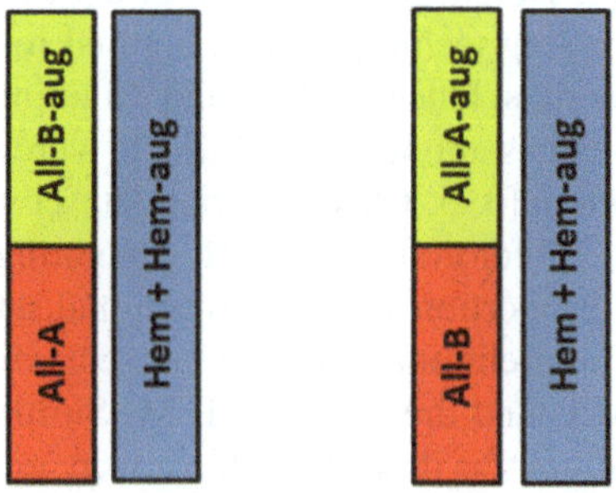

(a) Training set A (b) Training set B

Fig. 2 Composition of training sets

contrast, training set B consists of ALL samples from subset All-B and augmentation images from subset All-A. The HEM cells, as well as their augmentation part were employed in both training sets (A and B). Intuitively, each backbone model will "learn" the same HEM cell features but "mixed" ALL cell features from different compositions of All-A, All-B, and their image augmentation counterparts.

2.4 Training Strategy and "Combined" Model Architecture

Two-stage training strategy was employed in our experiments as described below for further increasing the overall model performance. For the first stage training, two Inception ResNets (denoted as model-A and model-B) with pre-trained ImageNet weights as initial were employed to be trained on the training set A and B, respectively. For the second stage training, models trained in the first stage were "combined" (see Fig. 3) and fine-tuned using all the ALL and HEM cells in the training set. In detail, the pretrained Inception ResNets in the first stage were employed as image features extractors. The outputs from penultimate layers (global average pooling layer, 1536-dim vector) from each Inception ResNet were concatenated after the batch normalization operation (not shown in Fig. 2 for simplicity) for reducing the influences of possible large magnitude differences between two output feature vectors from model-A and model-B. Next, two fully connected (FC, 1024 neurons each) layers with dropout operation (dropout rate = 0.6) were added to increase the prediction accuracy of the "combined" model. The output layer of the "combined" model was another FC layer with softmax activation function conventionally. This model, as its name showed, combines learned partial representative features from two ALL subsets and will further increase the prediction accuracy.

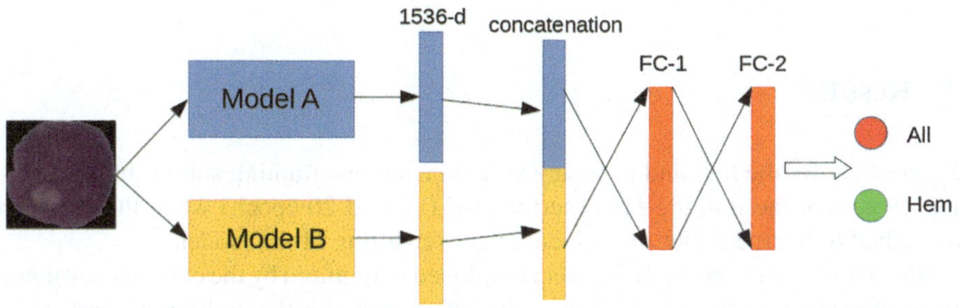

Fig. 3 Structure of the "combined" model

2.5 Training Settings

During training, RMSprop optimization [9] with all the settings default was employed. The total epochs were set to 50 empirically. In order to reduce the over-fitting and increase the performances of all models (model-A, model-B and "combined" one), several common training techniques were employed as followings shown. First, the validation error was calculated and monitored after each epoch during training. In our settings, the learning rate would be reduced with rate 0.1 after the validation error stagnated for 6 epochs. Besides training would be terminated if validation error stagnated for 12 epochs. Second, to the ALL and HEM cells discrimination, since the false-negative predictions generally cause higher risk than false-positive ones in clinical situations, herein, in order to reduce the false-negative rate, different class weights were applied to ALL cells and HEM cells empirically when optimizing loss function (Eq. 1) of "combined" model ($\lambda_{\text{All}} = 2.5$ for ALL cells and $\lambda_{\text{Hem}} = 1.0$ for HEM cells).

$$\mathcal{L}^{\text{total}} = \lambda_{\text{All}}\mathcal{L}^{\text{All}} + \lambda_{\text{Hem}}\mathcal{L}^{\text{Hem}} \tag{1}$$

All the training and validation operations were performed on one Ubuntu 16.04 server (with one GPU 1080), employing Keras (ver. 2.2.4) with Tensorflow (ver. 1.12.0) backend.

2.6 Inference

The final predictions were made using the combinations of Model A, B, and "combined" one. Specifically, the output prediction probabilities of each model for one sample were compared together and the label of the prediction which had the maximum probability was employed as the final result.

3 Results

Figure 4 shows the loss and accuracy variations on one training subset during training. Note that the training phase terminated (around 20 epoch) when the criterion described in Sect. 2.5 met for reducing the over-fitting of the model.

Precision, recall and F_1-score were employed as required by the contest to evaluate the performance of the model. Table 1 lists the results for the preliminary test set.

Due to the nature of the imbalanced preliminary test set, weighted average (support weighted mean per label) was also reported in Table 1. From the table, it is clear that the average prediction accuracy of ALL cells is higher than the one of HEM cells, which from the real clinical applications is more acceptable since mistakenly classifications of HEM cells to ALL cells suffer much lower risk than reversed predictions (ALL cells to HEM cells). The F_1-score of the final test set is 0.876.

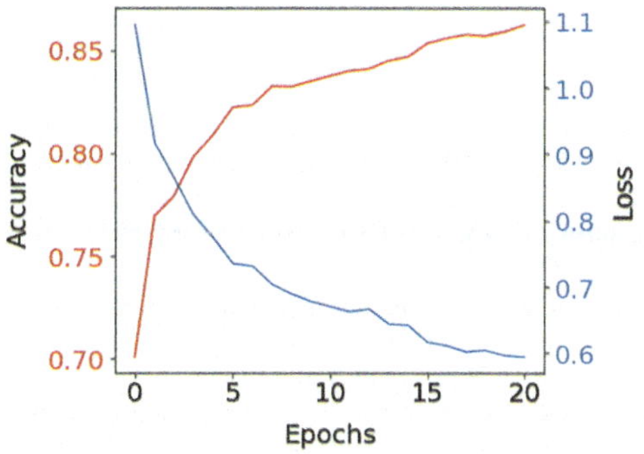

Fig. 4 Accuracy and loss of training subset during training phase

Table 1 Model performances of preliminary test set

Cell type	Precision	Recall	F_1-score	Support
Hem	0.80	0.74	0.77	648
All	0.87	0.90	0.88	1219
Weighted avg.	0.84	0.85	0.84	1867

4 Discussions and Conclusion

In the manuscript, we proposed a two-stage image augmented enhanced bagging ensemble training scheme to solve the classification of ALL cells and HEM cells. From the experiments, the training strategy, as well as elaborately designed training subsets, are efficient for tackling the challenges (deficient training samples and fine-grained image classification). One point needs to be noticed is that through our training parameters settings, less ALL cells prediction error is made compared with HEM cells. Also, we would like to point out that although utilizing the model ensemble strategy to increase the overall performance, our solution is lighter compared with the one employing multiple deep models to boost the accuracy, which is quite impractical in real situations due to higher model loading burden and longer prediction latency.

In the future, more training samples are necessary to further increase the overall performance of model predictions. Besides, the blood cell detection from the scanned images should be included to make the whole procedure pragmatic. Finally, the efficiency of DL based ALL cell image analysis has to be validated with real clinical environments, not this kind of well-defined contest.

References

1. Disease, G., Incidence, I., Collaborators, P.: Global, regional, and national incidence, prevalence, and years lived with disability for 310 diseases and injuries, 1990–2015: a systematic analysis for the global burden of disease study 2015. Lancet (London, England) **388**(10053), 1545–1602 (2016). https://doi.org/10.1016/S0140-6736(16)31678-6. https://www.ncbi.nlm.nih.gov/pmc/articles/PMC5055577/
2. Duggal, R., Gupta, A., Gupta, R.: Segmentation of overlapping/touching white blood cell nuclei using artificial neural networks. In: CME Series on Hemato-Oncopathology, All India Institute of Medical Sciences (AIIMS). New Delhi, India (2016)
3. Duggal, R., Gupta, A., Gupta, R., Mallick, P.: SD-layer: stain deconvolutional layer for CNNs in medical microscopic imaging. In: Descoteaux, M., Maier-Hein, L., Franz, A., Jannin, P., Collins, D.L., Duchesne, S. (eds.) Medical Image Computing and Computer Assisted Intervention MICCAI 2017. Lecture Notes in Computer Science, pp. 435–443. Springer International Publishing (2017)
4. Duggal, R., Gupta, A., Gupta, R., Wadhwa, M., Ahuja, C.: Overlapping cell nuclei segmentation in microscopic images using deep belief networks. In: Proceedings of the Tenth Indian Conference on Computer Vision, Graphics and Image Processing, ICVGIP'16, pp. 82:1–82:8. ACM, Guwahati, Assam, India (2016). https://doi.org/10.1145/3009977.3010043
5. Gupta, A., Duggal, R., Gupta, R., Kumar, L., Thakkar, N., Satpathy, D.: GCTI-SN: geometry-inspired chemical and tissue invariant stain normalization of microscopic medical images (under review)
6. Gupta, R., Mallick, P., Duggal, R., Gupta, A., Sharma, O.: Stain color normalization and segmentation of plasma cells in microscopic images as a prelude to development of computer assisted automated disease diagnostic tool in multiple myeloma. Clin. Lymphoma, Myeloma Leuk. **17**(1), e99 (2017). https://doi.org/10.1016/j.clml.2017.03.178. https://www.clinical-lymphoma-myeloma-leukemia.com/article/S2152-2650(17)30468-8/abstract
7. Li, C.: Classifying imbalanced data using a bagging ensemble variation (BEV). In: Proceedings of the 45th Annual Southeast Regional Conference. pp. 203–208. ACM-SE 45, ACM (2007). https://doi.org/10.1145/1233341.1233378
8. Rehman, A., Abbas, N., Saba, T., Rahman, S.I.U., Mehmood, Z., Kolivand, H.: Classification of acute lymphoblastic leukemia using deep learning. Microsc. Res. Tech. **81**(11), 1310–1317 (2018). https://doi.org/10.1002/jemt.23139
9. Ruder, S.: An overview of gradient descent optimization algorithms (2016). arXiv:1609.04747 [cs]
10. Shafique, S., Tehsin, S.: Acute lymphoblastic leukemia detection and classification of its subtypes using pretrained deep convolutional neural networks. Technol. Cancer Res. Treat. **17** (2018). https://doi.org/10.1177/1533033818802789. https://www.ncbi.nlm.nih.gov/pmc/articles/PMC6161200/
11. Szegedy, C., Ioffe, S., Vanhoucke, V., Alemi, A.: Inception-v4, inception-ResNet and the impact of residual connections on learning. In: AAAI Conference on Artificial Intelligence (2017)
12. Tajbakhsh, N., Shin, J.Y., Gurudu, S.R., Hurst, R.T., Kendall, C.B., Gotway, M.B., Liang, J.: Convolutional neural networks for medical image analysis: full training or fine tuning? IEEE Trans. Med. Imag. **35**(5), 1299–1312 (2016). https://doi.org/10.1109/TMI.2016.2535302
13. Vununu, C., Lee, S.H., Kwon, K.R.: A deep feature extraction method for HEp-2 cell image classification. Electronics **8**(1), 20 (2019). https://doi.org/10.3390/electronics8010020. https://www.mdpi.com/2079-9292/8/1/20
14. Wang, Q., Wang, J., Zhou, M., Li, Q., Wang, Y.: Spectral-spatial feature-based neural network method for acute lymphoblastic leukemia cell identification via microscopic hyperspectral imaging technology. Biomed. Opt. Express **8**(6), 3017–3028 (2017). https://doi.org/10.1364/BOE.8.003017. https://www.ncbi.nlm.nih.gov/pmc/articles/PMC5480446/

15. Yu, L., Chen, H., Dou, Q., Qin, J., Wang, P.A.: Automated melanoma recognition in dermoscopy images via very deep residual networks. IEEE Trans. Med. Imag. **36**, 994–1004 (2017)
16. Zhang, J., Xie, Y., Wu, Q., Xia, Y.: Skin lesion classification in dermoscopy images using synergic deep learning. In: Medical Image Computing and Computer-Assisted Intervention-MICCAI 2018, vol. 11071, pp. 12–20 (2018)

Leukemic B-Lymphoblast Cell Detection with Monte Carlo Dropout Ensemble Models

Hao-Yu Yang and Lawrence H. Staib

Abstract Automatic detection of Leukemic B-lymphoblast cells from normal cells is both crucial and difficult with subject variability being a major obstacle. While deep learning models are widely adopted in image recognition and demonstrate state-of-the-art performance, deep learning models in their vanilla form do not provide an estimate of prediction uncertainty. This is especially problematic when there is a high discrepancy between training and testing data such as in blood smear images where subject level variability and sample noise from staining and illumination are non-negligible. To address these issues, we propose a novel ensemble method by weighting each base model according to its respective predictive confidence obtained from Monte Carlo dropout. Our ensemble method can effectively prevent overfitting and increases classification performance compared to any single model result. Furthermore, we demonstrate the model's ability to identify samples that do not fall in the training data distribution. We achieved 0.8929 prediction score according to the leaderboard on the SBILab challenge website.

Keywords Monte Carlo dropout · Model uncertainty · Ensemble model · Convolutional neural network

1 Introduction

Leukemia is a form of deadly cancer that causes the body's blood-forming tissue to generate malignant white blood cells. Most forms of leukemia such as Acute Lymphoblastic Leukemia (ALL) have no obvious symptoms in their early stages and

---

H.-Y. Yang (✉) · L. H. Staib
Yale University, New Haven, CT 06511, USA
e-mail: hao-yu.yang@yale.edu

L. H. Staib
e-mail: lawrence.staib@yale.edu

H.-Y. Yang
Cura Cloud Cooperation, Seattle, WA 98104, USA

A. Gupta and R. Gupta (eds.), *ISBI 2019 C-NMC Challenge: Classification in Cancer Cell Imaging*, Lecture Notes in Bioengineering,
https://doi.org/10.1007/978-981-15-0798-4_13

therefore, are often diagnosed during routine blood tests. Typical ALL diagnosis involves blood smears, which is the examination of stained blood under a microscope. A pathologist will then determine the malignancy of the blood samples based on the cell's appearance, size, and relative proportion. Machine-based classification of healthy and malignant white blood cell images presents high clinical value in low-cost diagnosis and early treatment. However, the problem is challenging due to several complications. First, malignant cells show similar morphological attributes with healthy cells. Second, intersubject variation is difficult to model with a conventional machine learning method. With the recent advances in computer vision and deep learning, massive attention has been drawn to applying Convolutional Neural Networks (CNN) to medical imaging. Although neural networks have demonstrated state-of-the-art performance in numerous tasks, the inability to capture prediction uncertainty is a major shortcoming. In the realm of machine learning and artificial intelligence, one is particularly interested in a model's predictive performance on unseen data. Given a test data point that lies outside of the training data distribution, a model should return an uncertain answer when forced to predict. However, previous research has shown that the probabilities generated by softmax functions, commonly seen at the end of a standard CNN workflow, cannot be interpreted as model confidence [4]. It has also been shown that a neural network with a dropout operation added before every weighted layer is equivalent to a Bayesian approximation of a Gaussian Process [11]. Monte Carlo dropout (MC dropout) has been proposed as a theoretically sound solution to represent model uncertainty.

In this paper, we present a novel method for predicting malignancy of white blood cells incorporating an ensemble of models and weighting by uncertainty. We finetuned numerous state-of-the-art CNN architectures on the 2019 ISBI C-NMC challenge dataset that were trained using ImageNet. These models include Progressive Neural Architecture Search (PNASnet) [10], Squeeze-and-Excitation Networks (SENet) [8], Inception Networks [12], DenseNet [9] and ResNet [7]. Model uncertainty was obtained by performing MC dropout during test time. The uncertainty information was then used for ensemble weighting of the aforementioned bag-of-models. Models with higher uncertainty are assigned fewer votes while higher confidence models have more voting power. The Monte Carlo dropout ensemble demonstrated a performance boost over single base learners. Furthermore, the uncertainty measure provides a robust metric for evaluating samples that the model finds uncertain.

2 Method

2.1 Data and Preprocessing

The proposed method (see Fig. 1) was trained, validated, and tested on the ISBI 2019 "Classification of Normal versus Malignant Cells in B-ALL White Blood Cancer Microscopic Images" challenge dataset [1–3, 5, 6]. The training dataset contains

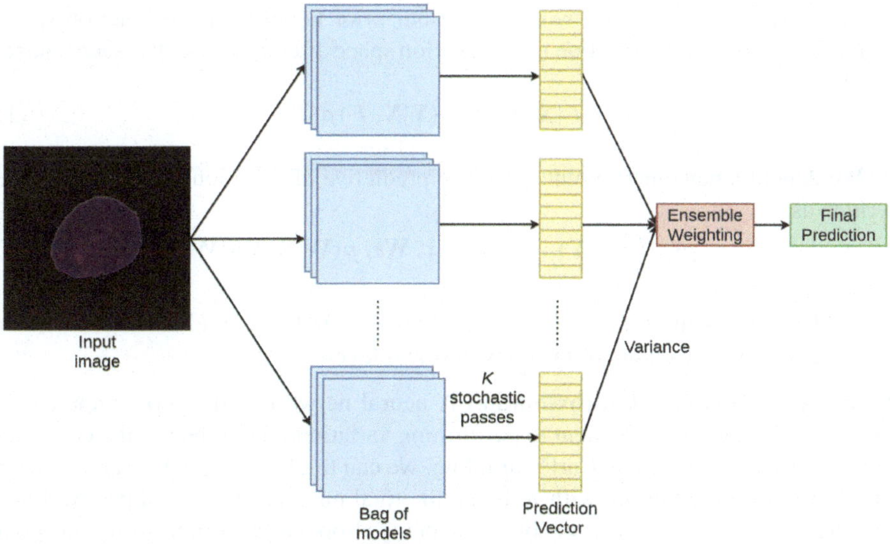

Fig. 1 Overview of the proposed Monte Carlo dropout ensemble method

samples from 76 individual subjects, 47 of which were diagnosed with cancer and the other 29 were healthy. A single-subject has multiple cell images. There are 7272 cancerous cell images and 3389 normal cell images totaling 10,661. The preliminary test set consisted of 1867 images from 30 subjects.

Data Imbalance The dataset is imbalanced in that the malignant cell images outnumber the normal cell images roughly 2–1. To overcome this issue, we sampled normal cell images twice as much as malignant cell images.

Data Augmentation For preprocessing and data augmentation, images were randomly cropped, scaled, and resized to 450 by 450 pixels during training. We also applied a random affine transformation, horizontal and vertical flip, and random adjustments, in contrast, brightness and saturation by 0.05.

2.2 Monte Carlo Dropout

In this section, we briefly discuss the necessary statistical tools, such as the Gaussian process, for the foundation of Monte Carlo dropout. Then we present our ensemble methods based on the uncertainty metric obtained from Monte Carlo dropout.

Gaussian Process A Gaussian process is a member of a broader family of statistical tools denoted nonparametric Bayesian inference. It is often used to model the distribution over functions by placing prior beliefs about the function on an infinite dimensional space.

In a Bayesian setting, we would place our prior belief over the function space $p(F)$. The posterior distribution is the function space after the model has seen dataset $(\mathbf{X}, \mathbf{Y})$:

$$p(F|\mathbf{X}, \mathbf{Y}) \propto p(\mathbf{Y}|\mathbf{X}, F)p(F) \tag{1}$$

We denote a new query point as $\hat{x}$. The predictive distribution can, therefore, be written as:

$$p(\hat{y}|\hat{x}, \mathbf{X}, \mathbf{Y}) = \int p(\hat{y}|\hat{x}, \mathbf{W}), p(\mathbf{W}|\mathbf{X}, \mathbf{Y})d\mathbf{W} \tag{2}$$

where $\mathbf{W}$ denotes the set of random variables the model is conditioned on. In our case, these are the weights of the convolutional layers.

Dropout as Bayesian Approximation A neural network with dropout applied at every weight layer is equivalent to performing variational inference of the Gaussian process. To perform Monte Carlo sampling, we can think of dropout as a realization of a Bernoulli distribution, with K being the total number of forward passes. Each weighted parameter has a probability of being dropped according to the dropout rate that is set. The expected value of the approximate predictive distribution can be written as:

$$\mathbb{E}_{q(\hat{y}|\hat{x})(\hat{y})} \sim \frac{1}{K}\sum_{k=1}^{K} \hat{y}(\hat{x}, \mathbf{W}_1^k, \ldots, \mathbf{W}_L^k) \tag{3}$$

2.3 *Ensemble by Uncertainty*

Ensemble learning involves combining multiple base learners with a meta-algorithm to form an ensemble model. Typically, ensembling models offer better generalization than the base learners. Since the true function of interest might not lie in the hypothesis space that is being searched, ensemble models with different hypothesis spaces can offer a better approximation of the true function. We present our ensemble algorithm in Algorithm 1.

Algorithm 1: Monte Carlo Dropout ensemble

Require: *Trained Base models* $\mathcal{M}_1 \ldots \mathcal{M}_\mathcal{L}$
Data: query point $\hat{x}$
for $\mathcal{M}_1$ *to* $\mathcal{M}_\mathcal{L}$ **do**
    for i = *1 to T* **do**
        $\hat{y}_i \leftarrow \mathcal{M}(\hat{x})$
    end
end

We denote the uncertainty of a single model $\mathcal{M}_l$ predicting on query point $\hat{x}$ as $\text{Var}(\mathcal{M}_l(\hat{x}))$, which can be calculated with the following:

$$\text{Var}(\mathcal{M}_l(\hat{x})) = \frac{\sum_{t=1}^{T}(\hat{y}_t - \bar{y})^2}{T} \quad (4)$$

where $\hat{y}_t$ denotes the prediction result on the tth pass and $\bar{y}$ is the average softmax output across all T passes. The weighting coefficient λ_l assigns uncertain models with less votes and certain models more votes:

$$\lambda_l = \frac{\sum_{l=1}^{L} \text{Var}(\mathcal{M}_l(\hat{x}))}{\text{Var}(\mathcal{M}_l(\hat{x}))} \quad (5)$$

Finally, the ensemble results are conducted by majority voting with:

$$\hat{y} = \text{mode}\{\lambda_1 \bar{y}_1, \ldots, \lambda_L \bar{y}_L)\} \quad (6)$$

2.4 *Implementation Details*

All code was developed with Python under the PyTorch deep learning framework. GPU training was conducted on an NVIDIA Tesla V100. The initial training rate was set at 0.001 and the learning rate decay at 0.0001. We used a batch size of 32. We have experimented with 10, 100, 1000 stochastic forward passes of Monte Carlo dropout and find that 100 passes are the best for trading off efficiency and performance.

3 Results

Below we discuss the effects of Monte Carlo dropout and report the preliminary test set performance across our bags of base models and ensemble results on the ISBI C-NMC challenge dataset.

Monte Carlo Dropout Results We perform Monte Carlo dropout with 100 stochastic forward passes on the preliminary test set. Figure 2 shows samples with the highest and lowest uncertainty from InceptionResnetV2 and InceptionV4 [12] predicting on the preliminary test set. It can be seen that samples with high uncertainty involved some morphological irregularities from the general training distribution, i.e., connected cells in the same image or cutoff artifacts. The two models showed similar behavior and performance.

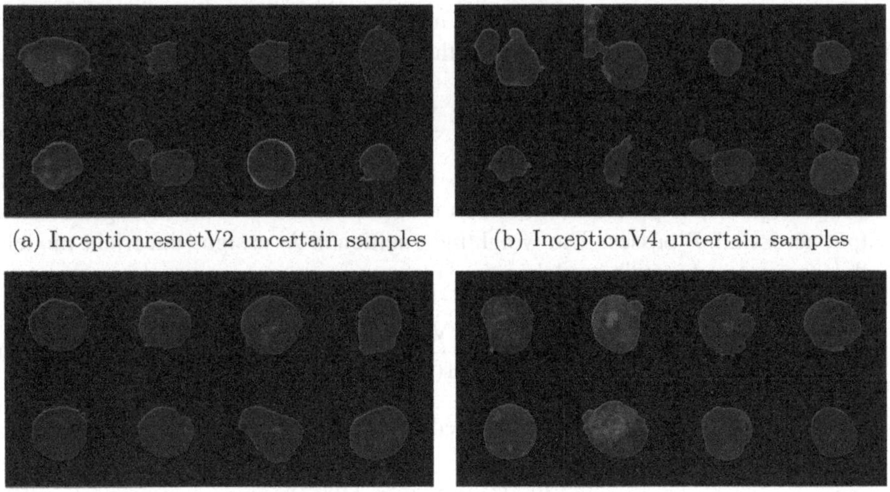

(a) InceptionresnetV2 uncertain samples (b) InceptionV4 uncertain samples

(c) InceptionresnetV2 certain samples (d) InceptionV4 certain samples

Fig. 2 Certain and uncertain samples from InceptionV4 and InceptionResnetV2

Table 1 Performance on the ISBI C-NMC preliminary test set results

Base models	Average uncertainty	F1 score
ResNet152	0.0335	0.756
DenseNet161	0.0316	0.806
DenseNet201	0.00928	0.835
InceptionResnetV2	0.00068	0.884
InceptionV4	0.00752	0.850
SE ResNext 101 32 X 4d	0.00875	0.880
SE Net 154	0.0142	0.755
PNAS net	0.0167	0.821
Poly net	0.0152	0.839
NAS net	0.0178	0.820
Uncertainty ensemble	N/A	0.8929

ISBI C-NMC Preliminary Test Set Results We present the performance of each base learners and ensemble results on the ISBI C-NMC preliminary test set results in Table 1. Since we do not have the ground truth for the final test set results, we only present the ensemble results of 0.7486.

4 Discussion

We have proposed a novel method of ensemble models based on predictive confidence. The proposed model not only showed a performance boost that is otherwise unobtainable through a single base learner but more importantly offers a robust means of handling unseen data. We show that the uncertainty value obtained from Monte Carlo dropout reflects samples that each model finds uncertain. In imaging domains, such as blood smear microscopy, where illumination variation across subjects and staining errors are prevalent, an uncertainty metric is of key importance. The uncertain samples of each base model showed some overlap but most base learners have their own unique uncertain samples set. A small correlation of base learners is a desirable property for ensemble algorithms since the function space is enhanced. In future work, predictive confidence can also be used as a metric for active learning, where the model "picks" the most uncertain cases for expert clarification. The model will be initialized with a small training set and predict the rest of the data. The benefits of such a learning strategy include reducing the manual labeling effort by only annotating the most uncertain samples.

References

1. Duggal, R., Gupta, A., Gupta, R.: Segmentation of overlapping/touching white blood cell nuclei using artificial neural networks. CME Series on Hemato-Oncopathology (2016)
2. Duggal, R., Gupta, A., Gupta, R., Mallick, P.: SD-layer: stain deconvolutional layer for CNNs in medical microscopic imaging. In: Medical Image Computing and Computer-Assisted Intervention, MICCAI'17 (2017)
3. Duggal, R., Gupta, A., Gupta, R., Wadhwa, M., Ahuja, C.: Overlapping cell nuclei segmentation in microscopic images using deep belief networks. In: Indian Conference on Computer Vision, Graphics and Image Processing (ICVGIP) (2016)
4. Gal, Y., Ghahramani, Z.: Dropout as a Bayesian Approximation: Representing Model Uncertainty in Deep Learning (2015). arXiv:1506.02142
5. Gupta, A., Duggal, R., Gupta, R., Kumar, L., Thakkar, N., Satpathy, D.: GCTI-SN: geometry-inspired chemical and tissue invariant stain normalization of microscopic medical images. Under review
6. Gupta, R., Mallick, P., Duggal, R., Gupta, A., Sharma, O.: Stain color normalization and segmentation of plasma cells in microscopic images as a prelude to development of computer assisted automated disease diagnostic tool in multiple Myeloma. In: 16th International Myeloma Workshop (IMW), Mar 2017
7. He, K., Zhang, X., Ren, S., Sun, J.: Deep Residual Learning for Image Recognition (2015). arXiv:1512.03385
8. Hu, J., Shen, L., Albanie, S., Sun, G., Wu, E.: Squeeze-and-Excitation Networks (2017). arXiv:1709.01507
9. Huang, G., Liu, Z., van der Maaten, L., Weinberger, K.Q.: Densely Connected Convolutional Networks (2016). arXiv:1608.06993
10. Liu, C., Zoph, B., Shlens, J., Hua, W., Li, L., Fei-Fei, L., Yuille, A.L., Huang, J., Murphy, K.: Progressive neural architecture search. In: CoRR (2017). http://arxiv.org/abs/1712.00559

11. Rasmussen, C.E., Williams, C.K.I.: Gaussian Processes for Machine Learning (Adaptive Computation and Machine Learning). The MIT Press (2005)
12. Szegedy, C., Ioffe, S., Vanhoucke, V.: Inception-v4, inception-ResNet and the impact of residual connections on learning. In: CoRR (2016). http://arxiv.org/abs/1602.07261

ISBI Challenge 2019: Convolution Neural Networks for B-ALL Cell Classification

Ekansh Verma and Vijendra Singh

Abstract We Participated in International Symposium on Biomedical Imaging (ISBI) 2019 challenge: Classification of Normal versus Malignant Cells in B-ALL White Blood Cancer Microscopic Images. Acute Lymphoblastic Leukemia (ALL) is a cancer of the lymphoid line of blood cells characterized by the development of large numbers of immature lymphocytes. In this paper, we present a Convolutional Neural Networks (CNNs) based solution for the challenge. We designed our solution with pretrained MobileNetV2 architecture as base classifier. Also, we employ transfer learning as the amount of labeled data is limited and ensemble the trained base classifier variants to reduce the generalization error on prospective data. With our final solution we secured second place in the challenge with F1 score of 0.8947.

Keywords MobileNetV2 · White blood cancer · Convolutional neural networks (CNNs)

1 Introduction

Leukemia, also spelled as leukaemia, was the 13th most common cancer worldwide in 2018 [1]. In 2000, approximately 256,000 children and adults around the world developed a form of Leukemia, and 209,000 died from it [2]. In 2018, 437,033 new cases were diagnosed worldwide which contributes 2.6% of the total new cancer cases diagnosed (excluding non-melanoma skin cancer) worldwide [1]. Usually, repeated blood measure counts, and a bone marrow examination is used to diagnose leukemia when symptoms show up. In the early stages of the disease, blood tests may not show that person is leukemic. Advanced methods such as flow cytometry are available, but they are very expensive and are not widely used in pathology laboratories or hospitals,

E. Verma (✉)
Schlumberger Technology Center, Pune, India
e-mail: vermaekansh55@gmail.com

V. Singh
Robert Bosch Engineering and Business Solutions Private Limited, Bangalore, India
e-mail: vijendrasingh003@gmail.com

A. Gupta and R. Gupta (eds.), *ISBI 2019 C-NMC Challenge: Classification in Cancer Cell Imaging*, Lecture Notes in Bioengineering,
https://doi.org/10.1007/978-981-15-0798-4_14

particularly, in rural areas. Image analysis-based Computer-aided diagnosis (CAD) is emerging as new tool to diagnose such disease in cost-effective manner.

After the success of Convolutional Neural Networks (CNNs) in solving various pattern recognition based real-world problems [3], it is also seen as the most promising method in the field of medical image analysis. The performance of CNN based solutions depends on the availability of sufficiently large dataset. With the increase in diversity and availability of health care data, CNN can tackle more exciting medical image analysis problems. In this paper, we present an approach to classify malignant and benign white blood cancer cells using CNN.

We trained our model on the data provided under ISBI 2019 challenge: Classification of Normal versus Malignant Cells in B-ALL White Blood Cancer Microscopic Images. Given a "not very large" dataset (10,661), we used transfer learning so that we could start with a model that has already learned a lot of features from another large dataset. We trained different variations of pretrained MobileNetV2 [4] along with a few additional layers on the given dataset. In the end, ensemble of all the trained classifiers was used as final solution. The complete strategy is presented in detail under Sects. 3 and 4.

2 Data Description

Training phase data consists of 10,661 cell images in .bmp format out of which 7272 are malignant and 3389 are benign. Ground truth has been marked by the expert based on the domain knowledge. These cell images are distributed across 47 cancer affected subjects and 26 healthy subjects. These cells have been segmented from images of size 2560×1920 [5–7] after those images have been stain normalized [8, 9]. The resulting single-cell image is roughly the size of 300×300 pixels. As described in challenge, the images are representative of images in the real-world because these contain some staining noise and illumination errors, although these errors have largely been fixed by the organizers via their method of stain normalization. Besides the training set, the organizers provide a phase-2 dataset that includes 1,867 files. A number of malignant cells in phase-2 data are 1219 while rest 648 are normal. Phase 2 dataset is distributed across 13 cancer affected subjects and 15 healthy subjects. Additionally, test set with 2,586 cell images is provided by organizers for final evaluation.

3 Method

3.1 Data Preprocessing

Images provided for training and validation have a uniform size of 450×450. We crop training image of size 300×300 around center of the original image. Next, we

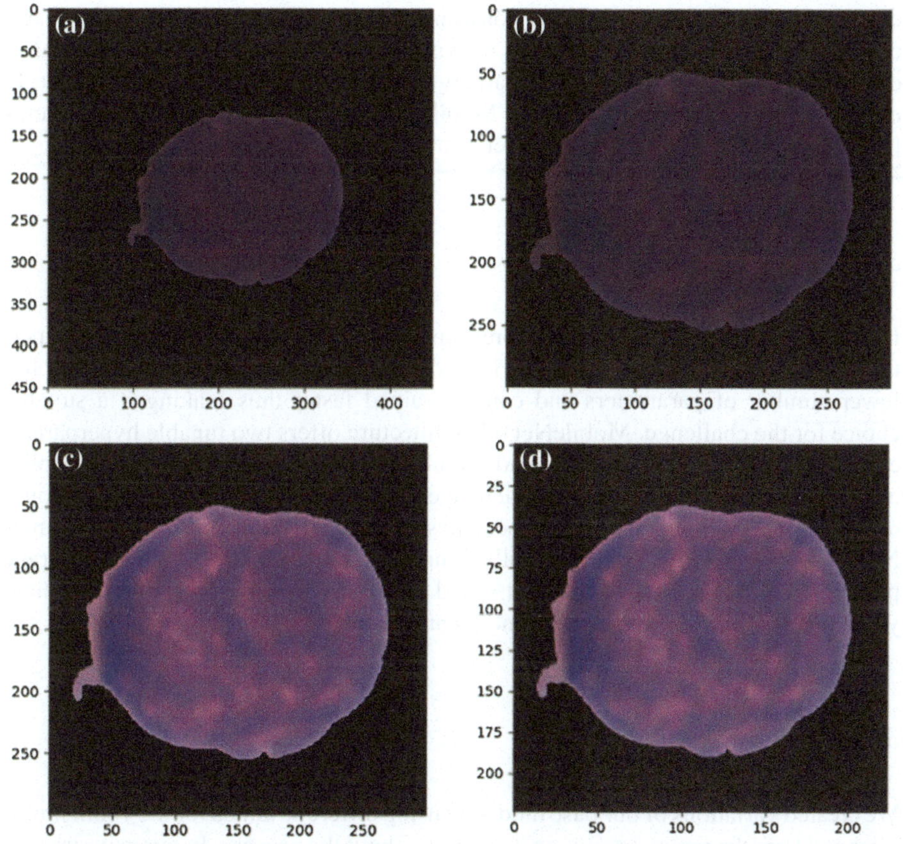

Fig. 1 **a** Original image, **b** cropped image, **c** normalized image, and **d** resized image

perform per image normalization as given in Eq. (1). Finally, we resize the image to 224 × 224 (Fig. 1).

$$I_{\text{norm}} = \frac{I - \min(I)}{\max(I) - \min(I)} \quad (1)$$

3.2 Transfer Learning

Transfer learning in deep learning refers to transferring knowledge from one domain to a similar one [10]. Due to the need for very large datasets, deep learning poses a challenge for medical applications. Thus, transfer learning becomes crucial for success. This is a common way to improve the performance of network on a smaller dataset by using a pretrained network on a larger dataset. Formally, we freeze the early convolutional layers of the proposed networks that are pretrained on the ImageNet dataset [11] and then retrain the remaining layers of the network on our dataset. In our experiments, we have chosen the MobileNetV2 model made available by Keras [12] which will be discussed in further sections.

3.3 Base Classifier

In our experiments, among all the pretrained models we tried, MobileNetV2 performed relatively better on the provided dataset. On top of it, MobileNetV2 has fewer number of parameters and can be trained faster thus making it a suitable choice for the challenge. MobileNetV2 architecture offers two tunable hyperparameters: input image resolution and width multiplier. The role of the width multiplier α is to thin a network uniformly at each layer. For a given layer and width multiplier α, the number of input channels M becomes αM and the number of output channels N becomes αN. We discarded the fully connected layer and added a global average pooling layer followed by dropout [13] and a dense layer with sigmoid activation to yield a probability score. The base model architecture is shown in Fig. 2.

3.4 Base Classifier Variants

We created variations of our base model by using different values for the width multiplier and kept the image resolution same throughout the process. In our experiments, reducing width multiplier increases the bias but decreases the variance of model hence we chose one variant with value of width multiplier 0.75. We experimented with the number of convolution layers to be frozen from top due to overfitting concerns and trained the remaining layers. Freezing the layers reduces the number of trainable parameters for our network. We decided to freeze first conv2d block and next nine inverted residual blocks of MobileNetV2. Finally, we had four networks varying in terms of width multiplier and the number of frozen layers (Table 1).

4 Experimental Settings

There is an imbalance between the images on subject level across malignant and benign class and as per challenge description subject level variability also plays a key role because of which it is difficult to build a classifier that can yield good results on prospective data. To overcome the challenge of imbalanced data and subject level variability we did subject wise K-fold cross-validation. We group the data by subject

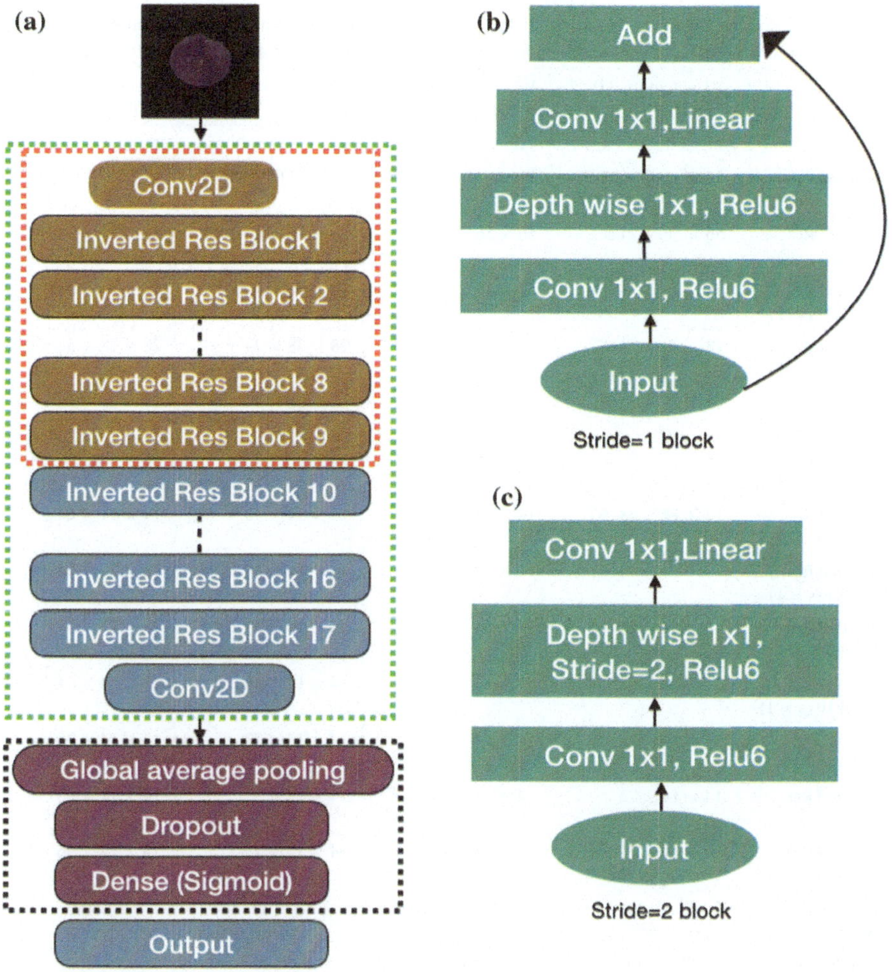

Fig. 2 Base model architecture. **a** Complete model architecture, blocks under green dotted rectangle is taken from MobileNetV2, blocks under red dotted rectangle has been frozen in some variants, and blocks under black dotted box are added over MobileNetV2 block, **b** inverted residual block with stride 1, **c** inverted residual block with stride 2

ID for both the classes. Next, we took 80% of total number of subject IDs in each class as training set and remaining as validation set.

The parameters were learnt by minimizing weighted binary cross-entropy loss with ADAM as the optimizer. Weighted binary loss implies that we give more weightage to the underrepresented class in vanilla binary cross-entropy function. The learning rate of ADAM was initialized to 10^{-3} and the learning rate was reduced by a factor of 10% if the monitored validation loss doesn't decrease. If validation loss does

Table 1 Model architecture of selected four variants, α shows width multiplier and f shows the number of fixed layers, output with (F) are the layer which has been frozen while training

Operator	V1 output (α = 0.75, f = 10)	V2 output (α = 1, f = 10)	V3 output (α = 0.75, f = 0)	V4 output (α = 1, f = 0)
Conv2d	112 × 112 × 24 (F)	112 × 112 × 24 (F)	112 × 112 × 2	112 × 112 × 24
Inverted Res Block1 (s = 1)	112 × 112 × 16 (F)	112 × 112 × 16 (F)	112 × 112 × 16	112 × 112 × 16
Inverted Res Block2 (s = 2)	56 × 56 × 24 (F)	56 × 56 × 24 (F)	56 × 56 × 24	56 × 56 × 24
Inverted Res Block3 (s = 1)	56 × 56 × 24 (F)	56 × 56 × 24 (F)	56 × 56 × 24	56 × 56 × 24
Inverted Res Block4 (s = 2)	28 × 28 × 24 (F)	28 × 28 × 32 (F)	28 × 28 × 24	28 × 28 × 32
Inverted Res Block5 (s = 1)	28 × 28 × 24 (F)	28 × 28 × 32 (F)	28 × 28 × 24	28 × 28 × 32
Inverted Res Block6 (s = 1)	28 × 28 × 24 (F)	28 × 28 × 32 (F)	28 × 28 × 24	28 × 28 × 32
Inverted Res Block7 (s = 2)	14 × 14 × 48 (F)	14 × 14 × 64 (F)	14 × 14 × 48	14 × 14 × 64
Inverted Res Block8 (s = 1)	14 × 14 × 48 (F)	14 × 14 × 64 (F)	14 × 14 × 48	14 × 14 × 64
Inverted Res Block9 (s = 1)	14 × 14 × 48 (F)	14 × 14 × 64 (F)	14 × 14 × 48	14 × 14 × 64
Inverted Res Block10 (s = 1)	14 × 14 × 48	14 × 14 × 64	14 × 14 × 48	14 × 14 × 64
Inverted Res Block11 (s = 1)	14 × 14 × 72	14 × 14 × 96	14 × 14 × 72	14 × 14 × 96
Inverted Res Block12 (s = 1)	14 × 14 × 72	14 × 14 × 96	14 × 14 × 72	14 × 14 × 96
Inverted Res Block13 (s = 1)	14 × 14 × 72	14 × 14 × 96	14 × 14 × 72	14 × 14 × 96
Inverted Res Block14 (s = 2)	7 × 7 × 120	7 × 7 × 160	7 × 7 × 120	7 × 7 × 160
Inverted Res Block15 (s = 1)	7 × 7 × 120	7 × 7 × 160	7 × 7 × 120	7 × 7 × 160
Inverted Res Block16 (s = 1)	7 × 7 × 120	7 × 7 × 160	7 × 7 × 120	7 × 7 × 160
Inverted Res Block17 (s = 1)	7 × 7 × 240	7 × 7 × 320	7 × 7 × 240	7 × 7 × 320
Conv2d 1X1	7 × 7 × 1280	7 × 7 × 1280	7 × 7 × 1280	7 × 7 × 1280
Global average pooling	1280	1280	1280	1280
Conv2d 1X1	1	1	1	1

not improve for predetermined number of epochs, training is stopped. We restore the model weights from the epoch with the lowest value of validation loss for inference.

The evaluation metric used throughout the challenge is F1 score as given in Eq. (2). It is defined as the harmonic mean of precision and recall. Precision is the ratio of true positives to the sum of true positives and false positives whereas recall is the ratio of true positives to the sum of true positives and false negatives.

$$\text{F1 score} = \frac{2 * \text{precision} * \text{recall}}{\text{precision} + \text{recall}} \tag{2}$$

We trained the four variants discussed above with 10-fold subject wise cross-validation. We selected models for ensemble by checking the drop in corresponding validation loss per epoch during training. In addition, we only retained the models which achieved F1 score greater than 0.80 on the internal validation set. Following this selection procedure, we ended up with a total of 13 models for our final ensemble. We worked on creating the meta-models but to us they appeared to be overfitting for the task and thus, we ended up using simple average probabilities ensemble for final prediction.

5 Results and Discussion

Our ensemble of classifiers achieved 0.87025 F1 scores on the held out phase 2 test dataset. With model ensemble we achieved an improvement of 3.3% in F1 score on phase 2 dataset when compared to our top-performing model variant.

The number of malignant cells in phase-2 data is 1219 while rest 648 is normal. Phase 2 dataset is distributed across 13 cancer affected subjects and 15 healthy subjects. We report the result of our proposed solution on phase 2 test data both class and subject wise in Figs. 3 and 4, respectively. On final test data our solution achieves 0.8947 F1 scores and ranks second on the final leaderboard.

6 Conclusion

We used MobileNetV2 as our base classifier and ensemble different variation of base classifier to form our final solution. We observed that ensemble of models improved the classification performance when compared to using a single model. Also compared to using all the models in ensemble our selection procedure of the models helps in achieving better F1 score. Transfer learning helped to a great extent in overcoming the unavailability of large datasets.

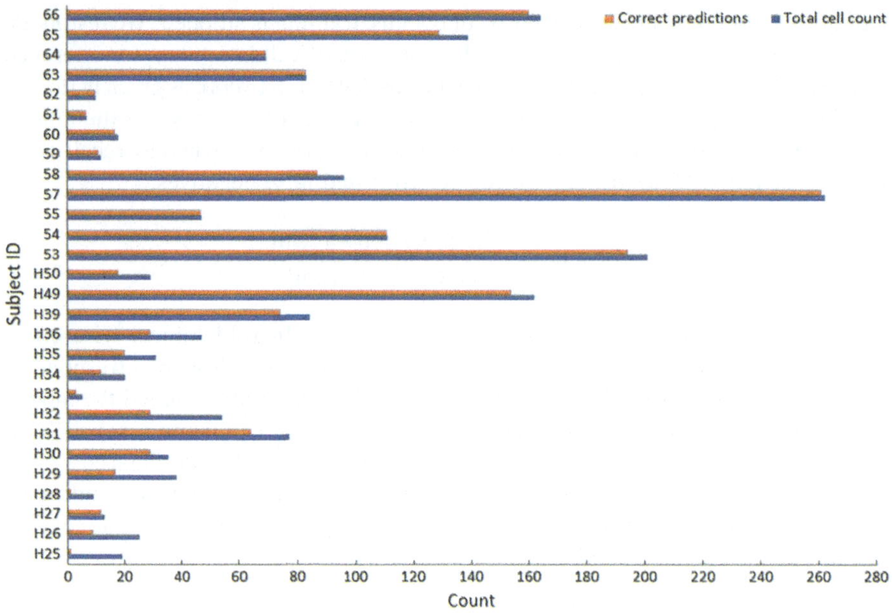

Fig. 3 Subject wise performance on phase 2 data. Subject with prefix 'H' is healthy and subject without any prefix are the patient with cancer

	Predicted Normal	Predicted Malignant
Actual Normal	472	176
Actual Malignant	60	1159

Fig. 4 Confusion matrix on phase 2 test data

References

1. Bray, F., Ferlay, J., Soerjomataram, I., Siegel, R.L., Torre, L.A., Jemal, A.: Global cancer statistics 2018: GLOBOCAN estimates of incidence and mortality worldwide for 36 cancers in 185 countries. CA Cancer J. Clin.
2. Mathers, C.D., Boschi-Pinto, C., Lopez, A.D., Murray, C.J.L.: Cancer incidence, mortality and survival by site for 14 regions of the world. In: Global Programme on Evidence for Health Policy Discussion Paper No. 13. World Health Organisation (2001)
3. Hinton, G.E., Krizhevsky, A., Sutskever, I.: Imagenet classification with deep convolutional neural networks. In: Advances in Neural Information Processing Systems, pp. 1097–1105 (2012)
4. Sandler, M., Howard, A., Zhu, M., Zhmoginov, A., Chen, L.C.: Inverted residuals and linear bottlenecks: Mobile networks for classification, detection and segmentation (2018). arXiv: 1801.04381

5. Duggal, R., Gupta, A., Gupta, R., Wadhwa, M., Ahuja, C.: Overlapping cell nuclei segmentation in microscopic images using deep belief networks. In: Indian Conference on Computer Vision, Graphics and Image Processing (ICVGIP), India, December 2016
6. Duggal, R., Gupta, A., Gupta, R.: Segmentation of overlapping/touching white blood cell nuclei using artificial neural networks. CME Series on Hemato-Oncopathology, All India Institute of Medical Sciences (AIIMS), New Delhi, India, July 2016
7. Duggal, R., Gupta, A., Gupta, R., Mallick, P.: SD-layer: stain deconvolutional layer for CNNs in medical microscopic imaging. In: Descoteaux, M., Maier-Hein, L., Franz, A., Jannin, P., Collins, D., Duchesne, S. (eds.) Medical Image Computing and Computer-Assisted Intervention-MICCAI 2017. Lecture Notes in Computer Science, Part III, LNCS 10435, pp. 435–443. Springer, Cham (2017)
8. Gupta, A., Duggal, R., Gupta, R., Kumar, L., Thakkar, N., Satpathy, D.: GCTI-SN: geometry-inspired chemical and tissue invariant stain normalization of microscopic medical images
9. Gupta, R., Mallick, P., Duggal, R., Gupta, A., Sharma, O.: Stain color normalization and segmentation of plasma cells in microscopic images as a prelude to development of computer assisted automated disease diagnostic tool in multiple myeloma. In: 16th International Myeloma Workshop (IMW), India, March 2017
10. Bengio, Y.: Deep learning of representations for unsupervised and transfer learning. In: Proceedings of ICML Workshop on Unsupervised and Transfer Learning, pp. 17–36 (2012)
11. Deng, J., Dong, W., Socher, R., Li, L.-J., Li, K., Fei-Fei, L.: ImageNet: a large-scale hierarchical image database. In: CVPR09 (2009)
12. Chollet, F. (2015) keras, GitHub. https://github.com/fchollet/keras
13. Srivastava, N., Hinton, G., Krizhevsky, A., Sutskever, I., Salakhutdinov, R.: Dropout: a simple way to prevent neural networks from overfitting. JMLR (2014)

Classification of Cancer Microscopic Images via Convolutional Neural Networks

Mohammad Azam Khan and Jaegul Choo

Abstract This paper describes our approach for the classification of normal versus malignant cells in B-ALL white blood cancer microscopic images: ISBI 2019—classification of leukemic B-lymphoblast cells from normal B-lymphoid precursors from blood smear microscopic images. We leverage a state of the art convolutional neural network pretrained with the ImageNet dataset and applied several data augmentation and hyperparameters optimization strategies. Our method obtains an F1 score of 0.83 for the final test set in the competition.

Keywords B-lymphoblast cell · Blood smear · B-lymphoid · Blood cancer · Convolutional neural networks

1 Introduction

Automating the process of cell identification and segmentation has recently gained interest for building computer-assisted diagnostic tools. These tools can be very helpful in analyzing medical images for cell classification tasks containing blood disorders such as leukemia. In this concern, the C-NMC 2019 challenge [6] aims to build an automated classifier using different image processing tools. A robust classifier will assist pathologists and oncologists to make faster and data-driven inferences. In addition, the organizers have attempted to overcome the issues associated with deploying sophisticated high-end machines for medical image processing with recurring reagent costs through this competition.

This is unchallenged by now that convolutional neural networks (CNNs) dictate the state of the art in biomedical image processing. As a consequence, many successful CNNs are being used differently in medical imaging tasks including

M. A. Khan · J. Choo (✉)
Korea University, Seoul 136-713, South Korea
e-mail: jchoo@korea.ac.kr

M. A. Khan
e-mail: a_khanss@korea.ac.kr

A. Gupta and R. Gupta (eds.), *ISBI 2019 C-NMC Challenge: Classification in Cancer Cell Imaging*, Lecture Notes in Bioengineering,
https://doi.org/10.1007/978-981-15-0798-4_15

classification, segmentation, and so on [1, 12, 14, 16]. In this work, we used a state of the art network to classify normal versus malignant cells in B-ALL white blood cancer microscopic images in an end to end settings.

2 Dataset

The dataset [15] consists of cells with labels (normal versus malignant) to identify normal cells from leukemic blasts (malignant cells). Both the training and testing (preliminary and final) data contain subject and image level information. However, the dataset is imbalanced and the number of images for cancer class is almost double compared to its counter part normal (healthy) images for the both levels. The distribution of training and testing images are shown in Table 1.

3 Methods

Given a set of images, the goal is to automatically identify normal cells from leukemic blasts (malignant cells) in each image. In this section, we describe our preprocessing steps, data augmentation mechanism, and training procedure subsequently.

3.1 Data Preprocessing

The data is already preprocessed by the organizer. The images are representative of images in the real-world because these contain some staining noise and illumination errors. However, these errors have largely been fixed by the organizers via their inhouse method on stain normalization [2–4, 7, 8]. Nonetheless, each image contains a significant portion of black part which can be considered as background noise. As a further preprocessing step, we try to consider center cropping of the image since the target portion is mainly found in the middle of the image. Figure 1 shows the cropped image (dotted green part) for training and testing set, respectively. Secondly, considering the nature of the task, subject-level information is crucial and thanks

Table 1 Dataset composition

Data subset	Subject level		Image level	
	All	Normal	All	Normal
Train set	47	26	7272	3389
Preliminary test set	13	15	1219	648
Final test set	9	8	–	–
Total	69	49	7920[a]	4608[a]

[a]Final test set information of image level is not available during the manuscript submission

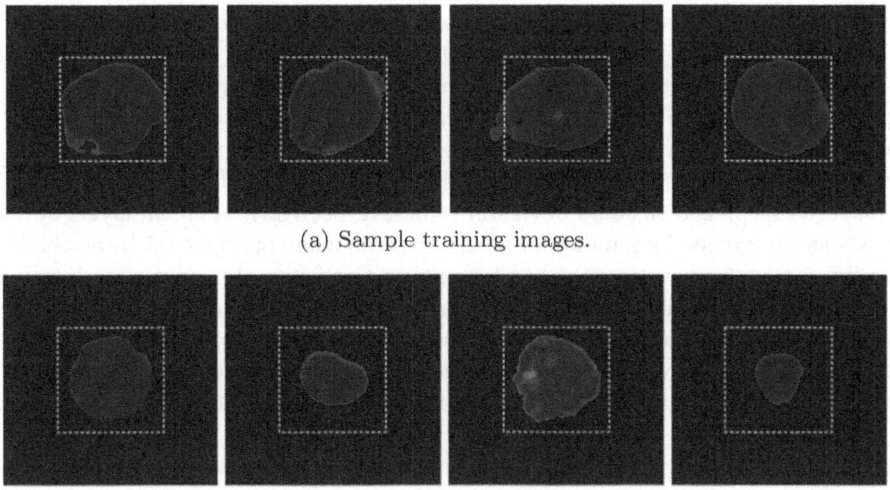

(a) Sample training images.

(b) Sample testing images.

Fig. 1 Cropping target part of the image to feed on the model

to the organizer for providing such information during the challenge period. The organizer also had made sure that subject level variability would play an important role while evaluation of the trained model on the test set. Considering the fact, we split the training and test set in such a way that no samples can be overlapped between the training and validation set.

3.2 Data Augmentation

The training set consists of 118 individual subjects in which cancer subjects are 69 and normal subjects are 49. We add all the possible ways of turning a square which is any combination of a horizontal flip, random rotations of 360°. This type of augmentation is somehow useful when we have satellite images, or derived from patches/images with nucleus/cells for instance.

3.3 Training

We tried mainly two popular CNN architectures for this task: ResNet [9] and its successor squeeze-and-excitation networks (SENets) [11] implemented in torchvision[1] and fine-tune pretrained Convolutional Neural Networks with PyTorch[2] with slight

[1]https://pytorch.org/docs/0.4.0/torchvision/models.html.

[2]https://github.com/creafz/pytorch-cnn-finetune.

architectural changes to fit our requirements. We replaced the final softmax layer with sigmoid one to cope up with our target task.

Previous work [5, 17] has shown that pretraining on a different domain improves performance. In addition, pretraining significantly improves convergence speed, so we use pretrained weight for initializing our model. An input image is normalized by channel-wise mean subtraction and divided by the standard deviation using ImageNet mean and standard deviation values, respectively. Then, all layers of our CNN are fine-tuned by training for 25 epochs with adam optimizer [13] (batches of 64 images) with an exponential-like learning rate policy: each 7 epochs the learning rate decreased by a factor of 10 (initially the learning rate was taken equal to 0.0001), and using the cross-entropy loss. We applied a data augmentation mechanism (at run time) by using horizontal flips and random rotations. Model selection was implemented by saving the network achieving the highest validation accuracy at the end of training.

It is worth noting that the dataset is partitioned into 6 subsets of approximately equal size. In addition, we utilize the preliminary test set as an additional set of training samples to develop our final prediction task.

4 Experimental Results

During the first phase of the competition, our approach was a bit different. We didn't try to make any preprocessing steps and attempted to train the model using the given images from low to higher resolution settings. However, training on higher resolution images, like 512×512, takes quite long time, and hence, training any model from scratch on such images is quite inefficient. Fortunately, modern convolutional neural nets support input images of arbitrary resolution. To decrease the training time, one can start training the model on low-resolution images first and then continue training on higher resolution images for only a few epochs. In addition, a model pretrained on low-resolution images first generalizes better since pixel information is less available and high order features are tended to be used.

Such functionalities are well implemented in most of the modern deep learning framework, however, our first choice was Fast.ai [10]. The head layers of the model are trained on 224×224 rescaled images for one epoch only. The following fine-tuning of entire model for 2 more epochs with learning rate annealing to boost up model performance. After that the training is continued for several epochs with a new/augmented data set composed of images of 384×384 resolution. Finally, we continue training the model on full resolution, 450×450. In this stage we reached a weighted F1-score of 0.8179 at the end of preliminary test phase. Model performance of different ResNet flavors is shown in Table 2.

The performance for the preliminary test set using our initial models was not good. Hence, we conducted experiments with several other state of the art neural networks. Among those, we selected SEResNets, a successor of universal network ResNet, due to its initial performance. This is a universal network which is extensively used mainly

Table 2 Performance of different ResNet models

Model	Validation F1-score	F1-score (online)
ResNet34	0.86	0.8036
ResNet50	0.86	0.7985
ResNet101	0.83	0.7851
Ensemble	0.84	0.8179

Table 3 Performance of final test set

Submission	Model	Validation F1-score	F1-score (online)
1	Ensemble	0.94	0.7839
2	SEResNet50	0.91	0.8317

for classification tasks. However, the model is also used as a feature extractor for encoder-decoder networks for segmentation tasks in addition to some other relevant tasks nowadays. Model performance of final test set is shown in Table 3.

5 Discussion

Our main intuition was to try how a single model may perform at most. Since the size of the images is relatively small, it is better to try early stage networks, such as ResNet34, VGGNet13, and so on. Occasionally, we conducted some experiments using state of the art deep or more stacked networks like ResNet101, DenseNet161, and VGGNet. However, the performance was not as good as their predecessor networks. The main reason behind this phenomenon is that early stage networks have sufficient capacity to work with low- resolution images. In addition we cropped target part of the images effectively and fed them into the model. This makes the image more smaller.

Unconsciously, we found a bug in our code after the maximum submission limit. The size of the image for training and preliminary test set was 450 × 450. However, for the final test set the image size was 600 × 600. So when we process center cropping based on the size 450 × 450, the target part was misleading for the final test set. Hence, our first ensemble submission performed worst and hence we were not able to utilize the second submission that much. We believe that our solution might perform better if we could utilize two submissions properly.

6 Conclusion

It is important to do early disease diagnosis for better cure and for improving the overall survival of the subjects suffering from cancer. In this work, we demonstrated that state of the art classification networks can be used for cell classification tasks effectively. We initially utilized the capacity of modern convolutional neural nets that support input images of arbitrary resolution, however, we finally concluded with a more generalized manner. All these mechanisms may be helpful to exploit for cell classification tasks. Such a fully automated method may hold great promise for increasing throughput and for aiding pathologists and oncologists to make quicker and data-driven inferences as well.

References

1. Christ, P.F., Ettlinger, F., Grün, F., Elshaer, M.E.A., Lipková, J., Schlecht, S., Ahmaddy, F., Tatavarty, S., Bickel, M., Bilic, P., Rempfler, M., Hofmann, F., D'Anastasi, M., Ahmadi, S.A., Kaissis, G., Holch, J.W., Sommer, W.H., Braren, R., Heinemann, V., Menze, B.H.: Automatic liver and tumor segmentation of CT and MRI volumes using cascaded fully convolutional neural networks. In: CoRR (2017). arXiv:1702.05970
2. Duggal, R., Gupta, A., Gupta, R.: Segmentation of overlapping/touching white blood cell nuclei using artificial neural networks (2016)
3. Duggal, R., Gupta, A., Gupta, R., Mallick, P.: SD-layer: stain deconvolutional layer for CNNs in medical microscopic imaging. In: Springer Proceedings in Physics, pp. 435–443. Springer, Singapore (2017). https://doi.org/10.1007/978-3-319-66179-7_50
4. Duggal, R., Gupta, A., Gupta, R., Wadhwa, M., Ahuja, C.: Overlapping cell nuclei segmentation in microscopic images using deep belief networks. In: Proceedings of the Tenth Indian Conference on Computer Vision, Graphics and Image Processing-ICVGIP. ACM Press (2016). https://doi.org/10.1145/3009977.3010043
5. Gulshan, V., Peng, L., Coram, M., Stumpe, M.C., Wu, D., Narayanaswamy, A., Venugopalan, S., Widner, K., Madams, T., Cuadros, J., Kim, R., Raman, R., Nelson, P.C., Mega, J.L., Webster, D.R.: Development and validation of a deep learning algorithm for detection of diabetic retinopathy in retinal fundus photographs. JAMA **316**(22), 2402 (2016). https://doi.org/10.1001/jama.2016.17216
6. Gupta, A., Gupta, R., Gehlot, S., Mourya, S.: Classification of normal vs malignant cells in B-ALL white blood cancer microscopic images. In: IEEE International Symposium on Biomedical Imaging (ISBI)-2019 Challenges Internet (2019). https://competitions.codalab.org/competitions/20395
7. Gupta, A., Duggal, R., Gupta, R., Kumar, L., Thakkar, N., Satpathy, D.: GCTI-SN: geometry-inspired chemical and tissue invariant stain normalization of microscopic medical images (under review)
8. Gupta, R., Mallick, P., Duggal, R., Gupta, A., Sharma, O.: Stain color normalization and segmentation of plasma cells in microscopic images as a prelude to development of computer assisted automated disease diagnostic tool in multiple myeloma. Clin. Lymphoma Myeloma Leuk. **17**(1), e99 (2017). https://doi.org/10.1016/j.clml.2017.03.178
9. He, K., Zhang, X., Ren, S., Sun, J.: Deep residual learning for image recognition. In: 2016 IEEE Conference on Computer Vision and Pattern Recognition (CVPR). IEEE (2016). https://doi.org/10.1109/cvpr.2016.90
10. Howard, J., et al.: fastai (2018). https://github.com/fastai/fastai

11. Hu, J., Shen, L., Sun, G.: Squeeze-and-excitation networks. In: 2018 IEEE/CVF Conference on Computer Vision and Pattern Recognition. IEEE (2018). https://doi.org/10.1109/cvpr.2018.00745
12. Johnson, J.W.: Adapting mask-RCNN for automatic nucleus segmentation (2018). arXiv:1805.00500
13. Kingma, D.P., Ba, J.: Adam: a method for stochastic optimization
14. Liu, Y., Gadepalli, K.K., Norouzi, M., Dahl, G., Kohlberger, T., Venugopalan, S., Boyko, A.S., Timofeev, A., Nelson, P.Q., Corrado, G., Hipp, J., Peng, L., Stumpe, M.: Detecting cancer metastases on gigapixel pathology images. In: MICCAI (2017). arXiv:1703.02442
15. Mourya, S., Kant, S., Kumar, P., Gupta, A., Gupta, R.: All Challenge Dataset of ISBI 2019 (2019). https://doi.org/10.7937/tcia.2019.dc64i46r
16. Prasoon, A., Petersen, K., Igel, C., Lauze, F., Dam, E., Nielsen, M.: Deep feature learning for knee cartilage segmentation using a triplanar convolutional neural network. In: Mori, K., Sakuma, I., Sato, Y., Barillot, C., Navab, N. (eds.) Medical Image Computing and Computer-Assisted Intervention-MICCAI 2013, pp. 246–253. Springer, Berlin, Heidelberg (2013)
17. Yosinski, J., Clune, J., Bengio, Y., Lipson, H.: How transferable are features in deep neural networks? In: Proceedings of the 27th International Conference on Neural Information Processing Systems, NIPS'14, vol. 2, pp. 3320–3328. MIT Press, Cambridge, MA, USA (2014). http://dl.acm.org/citation.cfm?id=2969033.2969197

The manufacturer's authorised representative in the EU is Springer Nature Customer Service Centre GmbH, Europaplatz 3, 69115 Heidelberg, Germany. If you have any concerns regarding our products, please contact ProductSafety@springernature.com

Printed and bound by CPI Group (UK) Ltd, Croydon, CR0 4YY
30/09/2026
02225465-0011